CLIMBING THE MOUNTAIN: CANCER, EXERCISE, AND WELL-BEING

Paul Stoller and Mitchell Stoller

Meyer & Meyer Sport

British Library Cataloguing in Publication Data
A catalogue record for this book is available from British Library

Paul Stoller and Mitchell Stoller:
Climbing the Mountain: Cancer, Exercise, and Well-being
Maidenhead: Meyer & Meyer Sport (UK) Ltd., 2014
ISBN: 978-1-78255-068-6

© 2015 by Meyer & Meyer Verlag, Aachen
Auckland, Beirut, Budapest, Cairo, Cape Town, Dubai, Indianapolis,
Kindberg, Maidenhead, Sydney, Olten, Singapore, Tehran, Toronto
Member of the World

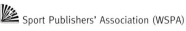 Sport Publishers' Association (WSPA)
www.w-s-p-a.org
Printing by: Print Consult GmbH, München
ISBN 978-1-78255-068-6
E-Mail: info@m-m-sports.com
www.m-m-sports.com

TABLE OF CONTENTS

ACKNOWLEDGEMENTS

ACKNOWLEDGMENTS

Writing a book is never a solitary enterprise. First and foremost, we thank Dr. Jasmin Tahmaseb McConatha, coeditor of this series of books on aging, health, and well-being, for suggesting that we write about cancer, exercise, and well-being. We also thank Dr. Karin Volkwein, another coeditor of the book series, for her enthusiastic encouragement. We would also like to thank Dr. McConatha for her thematic and editorial suggestions, which have helped us to fashion a draft into a clear, cohesive, and hopefully compelling text that will be useful to patients and families no matter their station on cancer's path.

We would also like to thank our families for their unflinching, ongoing support of our work in the world of cancer. They include Jasmin Tahmaseb, Lauren McConatha, Melina McConatha, Tim Spellman, Helena McConatha Rosle, Roxanne McConatha Spellman, Sheri Stoller, Betsy Stoller Davidian, Oren Davidian, Sam Davidian, and Lauren Stoller. Additionally, Paul Stoller would like to acknowledge West Chester University, where he has taught anthropology since 1980. Mitchell Stoller would like to acknowledge Dr. Margaret Foti and the American Association for Cancer Research (AACR), where he currently serves as Executive Director of the AACR Foundation.

PROLOGUE

PROLOGUE

Climbing a mountain is a challenge. For each of us the mountain looms in the distance among a patchwork of swirling dark clouds. The wind blows down from the partially obscured summit, suggesting that the path to the top may be fraught with difficulties—poor footing, steep inclines, slippery rocks, broken trails, sudden downpours, or precipitous drops in temperature. There are always many unknowns. Even so, most of us are willing and eager to risk discomfort and uncertainty as we set out on our hike up the mountain.

From where did this will to climb originate? Where did the will to risk uncertainty and potential danger come from? Long before we set foot on the mountain trail, we must commit to a regime of preparation. We invest in a pair of hiking boots, buy proper clothes, a windbreaker, and, of course, a hat. We also prepare our bodies for the physical challenges of mountain climbing, perhaps by lifting weights, jogging, and cycling to build stamina and help get us in shape. By the time we actually set foot on the trail, we are ready to face the challenge, anticipating the satisfaction of hopefully making it to the top, enjoying the view, and seeing the world from a new perspective.

Although not everyone has the inclination to climb an actual mountain, everyone confronts at least one existential mountain during his or her lifetime. The millions of people who are forced to face cancer are not unlike the hiker taking measure of his or her mountain. A cancer diagnosis looms like an unassailable peak, the immensity of which can be overpowering. How can we live with such a mortal challenge? How can we walk a trail that promises stress, fatigue, pain, and hair loss—a trail that is not likely to lead us to a majestic mountaintop? Cancer's trail often leads merely to remission—a respite, a way station on a path that may take to us to a sooner-than-expected death.

No matter where we live, a cancer diagnosis is the very antithesis of well-being; it is often a promise of misery and, for some people, a painful death. But this scenario is by no means preordained. With preparation and practice, the cancer patient, like the mountain hiker, can confront the challenges of a serious illness.

On this mountain trail, the cancer patient can move forward and upward on her or his path, taking calculated risks, adapting to the unevenness of the path, and most of all appreciating the trail's splendid views.

This book is about how cancer patients might prepare for their climb up the mountain. Although a cancer diagnosis will undeniably change a person's life, it should not be equated with a death sentence, even in the most severe circumstances. When we are coping with cancer, it is still possible to enjoy measures of well-being. This book reviews some of the challenges that cancer patients face.

The premise of the book is that one way to successfully adapt to the multiple constraints we face when we are diagnosed with cancer is to engage in preparation and practice. Preparation, as we suggest in this book, varies with our position on cancer's path. In the diagnostic stage, when uncertainty is at its highest point, research on potential treatment alternatives and reliance on the social support of friends, family, and colleagues is paramount. In the treatment stage, familiarizing ourselves with updated information about cancer and acquiring as much knowledge as possible about potential side effects, clinical trials, and new trends in clinical research is important. In periods of remission, awareness of ongoing research and social support continue to be vital to maintaining a degree of control and "normalcy" in life. No matter where we find ourselves on the path, exercising regularly, engaging in our hobbies, and continuing meaningful work and other activities can reduce the psychological stress and physical distress associated with cancer. Just as exercise can lead to feelings of well-being in the runner, swimmer, bicyclist, or mountain hiker, it can also enhance the cancer patient's sense of well-being.

This book is a user's guide to the cancer experience. In it we present a narrative of one cancer patient, John, who used preparation (research), practice (exercise and activity), and a variety of social supports to live "well" within the parameters that cancer imposed on his life. We also consider how the scope and patterns of preparation, practice, and social support change along cancer's trail. We discuss how to cope with the stresses and strains of diagnosis, treatment, and life in remission. In each chapter, we highlight the important relationships among exercise, activity, and well-being.

We follow this Prologue with **Part One**: Diagnosis, which consists of five chapters. In **Chapter 1**, we consider the challenge of confronting the possible diagnosis of a serious illness. How does a person deal with the existential uncertainty caused by such a diagnosis? In **Chapter 2**, we sound off about the ultrasound. An ultrasound is often an initial diagnostic test for potential cancers. What are its stresses and strains? Are there activities that can help us deal with such stress? **Chapter 3** is about the ins and outs of diagnostic CT and PET scans. These scans are used to detect enlarged lymph nodes, growing or shrinking tumors, or the biological presence of cancer cells. These procedures are, of course, stressful. What can we do to get through these ordeals? What role does exercise play? We consider doctor–patient relations in **Chapter 4**. We suggest that nothing is more important than establishing and maintaining rapport and trust with our oncologist. Is the oncologist "current?" Does he or she have a clinical or more humanistic approach to cancer care? What do our family members and friends think of the oncologist? How do we keep a clear head about our physician–patient relationship? In **Chapter 5**, we navigate the choppy waters of alternative cancer treatments. There are multiple choices on this path. How do we keep our heads straight when coming to a decision? Will our oncologist endorse complementary treatments like reflexology, massage, yoga, medication, and vitamin supplements? Will he or she respect our choices on the path to treatment?

In **Part Two**: Treatment, we present eight chapters that consider the whys and wherefores of cancer treatment. In **Chapter 6**, we consider the importance of our beliefs and of ritual practice during treatment. All human beings live in a particular culture. They are part of a culturally and socially conditioned system of beliefs. These beliefs and values shape people's views of illness, approaches to treatment, and post-treatment philosophies. All human beings engage in various rituals, which are structured behaviors that hold cultural and psychological meaning for participants.

Human beings perform rituals to gain a measure of control over an uncontrollable situation. Cancer treatments are fraught with stress and anxiety. One way of confronting uncomfortable and time-consuming chemotherapy or fearful radiation sessions is to construct a personal ritual that can be performed on each treatment visit. We also consider the role of camaraderie in the treatment room.

Treatment rooms can be spaces of social support and patient solidarity, which is a tonic for anyone going through chemotherapy. The central importance of nurse–patient relationships is considered in **Chapter 8**. During treatment, the rapport we establish with oncology nurses is essential to a positive and productive treatment experience. How can we establish good relations with our nurses? Why is such a relationship beneficial? In **Chapter 9**, we consider the benefits of treatment and post-treatment rituals like meditation.

While meditation is a good practice for anyone, not everyone is able to or has the desire to meditate. Studies have shown that meditation reduces stress and blood pressure. It centers our being and unclutters our minds, compelling us to discard stressful and unessential life elements and concentrate on what is important. It strengthens our psychological state and is a tonic to the immune system. It can give us a foundation of strength as we move through the long months of treatment. Meditation can be one helpful companion on our journey up the mountain.

Chapter 10 addresses the benefits of yoga. Like meditation, yoga practice reduces stress and increases physical flexibility. It enhances well-being and puts us in contact with other yoga practitioners who can provide social support. Yoga is another structured activity that guides us on our trail up the mountain. Both meditation and yoga are excellent activities for someone struggling with illness. They can be practiced at any level; even someone who feels weakened from treatment can reap benefits from meditation and yoga. Only five to ten minutes of yoga a day each can be helpful.

We explore reflexology and massage both during and after treatment in **Chapter 11**. The benefits of these practices are well known. They are increasing in popularity around the world. Both reduce stress, may bolster the immune system, and enhance well-being, all of which builds the fortitude to endure and overcome the emotional and physical side effects of cancer treatment. Throughout the book, but particularly in **Chapter 12**, we focus on the importance of social support during the cancer experience. Being a cancer patient is a lonely experience. Patients are better off if they confront the physical and psychological intangibles of cancer with the active support of family, friends, and fellow patients. Such support varies for each person. Support can take the form of conversations with intimate partners and close family, going to family gatherings, meeting with friends, and even participation in support groups. In the electronic age these resources have increased exponentially. Social support is now widely available through social media and Internet cancer support networks. In this book, we address the whys and wherefores of social support and discuss group activities that provide physical activity as well as social and emotional support.

In **Chapter 13**, we consider the possibility of post-treatment blues. Despite its stresses and strains, treatment routines can provide a measure of comfort to cancer patients. During the diagnosis phase, the uncertainty of our situation can be overwhelming. Do we actually have cancer? If so, what is our prognosis? How much time do we have left? Treatment is more concrete. We are taking steps to either cure or bring cancer into remission. We are working toward a goal. Time slows down. We take measure of our lives. When treatment comes to an end, we may even feel let down; we may feel that we are once again thrown back into uncertainty. Have we achieved our goal? What is next? How long will remission last? What happens if the cancer returns? Here, we focus on the importance of how physical and social activity can help us deal with post-treatment blues.

In **Part Three** of the book, we discuss remission, a stage of the cancer experience that researchers have insufficiently explored. When treatment ends and people enter remission, most think that they have survived the battle and have beaten the "beast" into submission. They may feel that they have climbed the mountain and made it to the summit. Remission, however, is not the end of the cancer experience. In **Chapter 14**, we explore the influence of indeterminacy during the remission phase. When treatment ends, we enter the world of remission, a world in which we are neither sick nor completely healthy. We may be symptom free, but we live with the knowledge that our cancer might return at any moment. Cancer has become a part of how we see ourselves and of how others see us. How can we cope with the existential uncertainty during remission? Remission is marked by indeterminacy. In such a space, which is between here and there, between past and present, between illness and health, we must make choices. Studies show that some people in remission fall into a state of deep depression and despair; others embrace the indeterminate period. Some people are able to embrace the possibilities they have been offered. They may use remission as a time of renewal, an exciting time of creativity, a time to refashion what is left of life. One way of embracing this indeterminate space is to be active—commune with nature, hike, take up gardening, learn a new skill, take on a new hobby, fulfill a long-held dream, and seek out the small pleasures of life.

In **Chapter 15**, we explore the importance of creativity. During remission, the ongoing practice of physical and mental exercise can trigger a multitude of creative outcomes that reinforce the resilience of the cancer patient. Studies have found that creative activities are linked to increased levels of well-being. In **Chapter 16**, we ponder the dynamics of well-being. What constitutes well-being? Can we measure it? What is its relationship to overall happiness? Is well-being long lasting or transitional? What role do preparation and practice play in cancer patients' quest for well-being? Do these help patients live more fully? How might focusing on strategies proposed in this book help cancer patients live happier lives?

In **Chapter 17**, we return to the practice of ritual during the post-treatment phase. With the right mix of preparation and practice, remission, which is usually symptom free, can be a time for living well in the world. But once or twice a year, the cancer patient must return to the world of medicine for a check-up, which usually involves an X-ray or CT scan to see if the cancer has returned. These routines are not at all routine. There is the build-up of tension prior to an office visit or scanning procedure. There is the possibility that our physician will feel something, perhaps a swollen lymph node, that shouldn't be there. When we go through these check-ups, the results might be positive, inconclusive, or negative. Based on these results, there may be an additional test or follow-up visits. Our oncologist might recommend another treatment regime. It is difficult to deal with these necessary procedures, but our lives depend on them. In this book, we address how we can cope with this complex and indeterminate phase of remission.

In the Epilogue of this book, we consider how cancer patients can live full lives. The world in which cancer patients live is different from the life lived by those who have not dwelled in the shadows of an incurable disease. For cancer patients the key is to be realistic about the possibilities but still manage to live fully and well within the parameters of our particular situations. A diagnosis of cancer is not an end to life, but the beginning of a new and different chapter of living in the world. It can be a life that is active and fulfilling. Through preparation, practice, active engagement, and support, it is a life that can be savored and lived fully, sometimes more fully than before the cancer diagnosis.

Resources for additional information on cancer research and survivorship:

American Association for Cancer Research:
www.aacrfoundation.org

LiveStrong Foundation:
www.LiveStrong.org

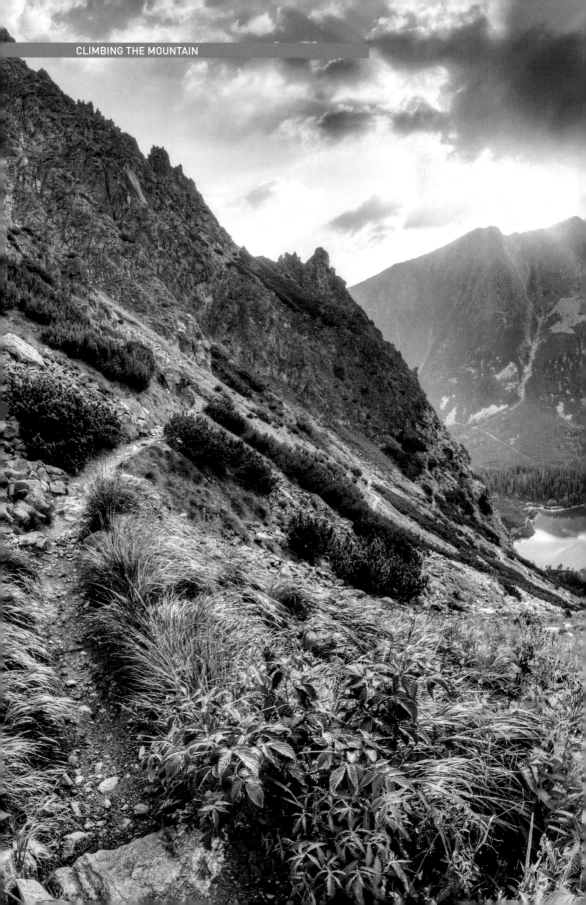

PART ONE

Diagnosis

PART ONE

Diagnosis

In this part of *Climbing the Mountain*, we discuss the frightening world of diagnosis. Diagnosis is a time (perhaps more than any other) filled with uncertainties. Until medical professionals are scientifically certain of the outcome of various diagnostic procedures, they are rightfully unwilling to say a person has a particular disease. Such professional vigilance, though important, can increase anxiety for patients waiting to hear if they have or do not have cancer. In the following chapters, we move through the various stages of cancer diagnosis, following the experiences of one cancer patient, John, through a matrix of procedures—medical examinations, ultrasounds, CT scans, and CT-scan-guided biopsies, as well as bone marrow biopsies.

John's case presents a particular set of medical and personal experiences; they vary for each individual. John's story represents the physical and emotional response of one person to the challenge of a potential cancer diagnosis and

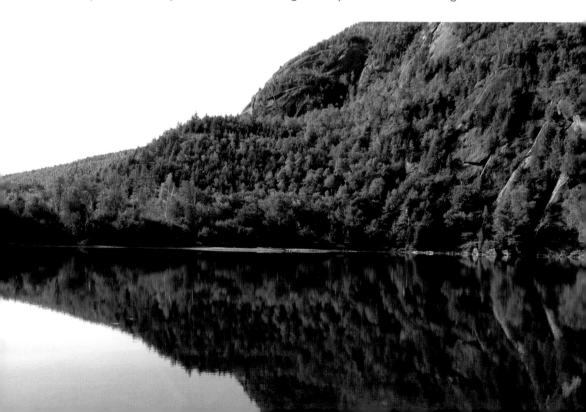

the necessity of choosing among treatment alternatives. There is no one way to proceed through the maze of diagnosis. In what follows, we tell John's story as a way to compel our readers to think about a variety of ways to cope with the uncertainties of diagnosis in the world of cancer.

1   CONFRONTING THE MOUNTAIN

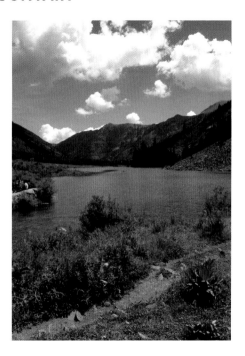

It's a beautiful spring day in 2012, and John, a tall, lanky, 50-year-old corporate lawyer, is on his way to his annual physical. If someone were to ask him about his life, he would say, "Life is good." He is a successful real estate attorney. He lives in a comfortable house in a quiet, woodsy suburb of Philadelphia, Pennsylvania. He's happily married to Beth, who is a social worker. They've been married for almost 20 years and have no children. They are comfortable enough financially to eat out when they want, go to concerts and plays, travel, and play golf.

John has always taken good care of himself. He eats a healthy diet of vegetables and consumes more fish than red meat. He drinks moderate amounts of wine, does not smoke, and makes time in his busy schedule to walk, hike, and ride his bicycle. These activities have kept him in good shape. John is easygoing and tends to be cheerful and optimistic. Though he has his worries, he has not thought much about his health. At his last physical, John's doctor said:

"You're in great shape, John. Whatever you're doing, keep doing it."

Driving to his physical and reflecting on life, John felt good about his situation—he was relatively prosperous, happy, and healthy. He didn't think too much about his physical. It was his turn to cook that night, which meant that he would have to stop at the market on the way home.

As the physical began, he felt little, if any, apprehension. He greeted his doctor, whom he had known for years. They chatted about the weather and their golf games. As they conversed, the doctor conducted his exam. John's lungs were clear, his reflexes were fine, his skin looked good, and his prostate was normal for his age. The doctor found no blood in his stool—a good sign. Then the doctor began to palpate John's abdomen and suddenly stopped.

"Let me feel that again," he said.

John's heart stopped, and he started feeling anxious. He began to focus on his physical. After more prodding, John's doctor told him that he had an abdominal mass, which might be nothing at all to worry about. But just to be safe, he ordered an ultrasound.

"Try not to worry," he told John. "It's probably nothing, but let's check it out."

Needless to say, John worried. He talked to Beth, and she worried. Whenever we have to check out a medical issue, it is worrisome. For the next two weeks, John went about his life with a new and unfamiliar sense of anxiety. Several days after the ultrasound, John went to see his doctor feeling considerably more trepidation than on his previous visits.

It appeared that his anxiety was well founded. The ultrasound revealed a large mass. John's doctor ordered a CT scan and set up an appointment with another physician, a medical oncologist. John could not believe that he was about to visit an oncologist's office. How did this happen? His initial check-up now seemed like the distant past. When the oncologist looked at John's scans, he suspected that his tumor might be malignant. He ordered a biopsy.

John had entered the world of diagnosis. The results of one test led to another. Throughout all of these procedures his life continued, but now John's life was filled with unwelcome anxiety. Sometimes he experienced his days more intensely than ever before. Sometimes it seemed that the whole day had been enshrouded in fog. Thankfully, Beth, his friends, and his co-workers were understanding and supportive.

The results of an unpleasant biopsy of his tumor confirmed the oncologist's suspicions. John had Non-Hodgkin Lymphoma (NHL). According to the World Health Organization (WHO), John's condition was one of 14 million new cancer cases in 2012 (http://www.who.int/mediacentre/factsheets/fs297/en/).

Like millions of other people, John would now have to undergo months of intensive cancer treatment. In what seemed like a split second, John's life had been turned upside down. His previous worries suddenly seemed inconsequential. He was facing entirely new challenges. The new path he was forced to take seemed perilous and steep.

THE CHALLENGE OF CHANGE

Everyone faces life-changing events. These events can be positive, such as winning the lottery, receiving an unexpected promotion, or falling in love. These positive events reinforce our love of life and perhaps our pre-existing sense of self. We savor the fact that our lives have been sweetened with good fortune.

Negative events are more challenging. When we confront the mountain of misfortune, we have to adapt to a set of sometimes unpleasant life circumstances. In addition, we usually have to adapt to these events quickly. Life-threatening conditions require immediate action. We need to make decisions about disease treatments, many of which will have significant, life-altering consequences. How will a treatment decision change our concept of self? How will we confront the physical and emotional suffering that invariably comes with long-term treatments for diseases like cancer? How will serious illness, which is for anyone a steep climb into the unknown, change our professional life? What kind of impact will it have on our families? Will they be able to accept our condition?

These first phases of the illness experience are perhaps the most stressful for patients confronting diseases like cancer. When we are in a space of existential uncertainty, like John, who for a few weeks did not know the details of his condition, it is difficult to know what to do. What if we have cancer? What if we don't have it? The worrisome possibilities are endless. We lose sleep. We may feel alone and isolated. Even if we are surrounded by loving family members, we often experience a profound loneliness.

How do we cope with this period of uncertainty?

No one likes to be situated in uncertain circumstances. Studies have demonstrated how to cope with the stress of uncertainty. There are a number of things we can do to reduce the stress of being in a place somewhere between health and serious illness.

SUGGESTIONS FOR COPING WITH THE EARLY STAGES OF A POTENTIAL CANCER DIAGNOSIS

1. **Try to carry on with your normal life.** Go to work. Try to keep professional and social appointments.
2. **Avoid rumination.** Try not to ruminate about your potential fate. Avoid sitting by your phone and waiting for the fateful call.
3. **Tap into nature's free therapy.** Find a park or a trail and take a leisurely or a vigorous walk in nature. Strolling among trees and listening to the gush of a stream's flowing waters takes you out of yourself, which has, for most people, a harmonious, calming effect. Or join a local hiking club through which you will enjoy nature's bounty as well as the enthusiastic camaraderie of fellow nature lovers.

4. **Make sure to exercise.** Exercise reduces anxiety and increases your feeling of well-being, which impels you to think about things other than your potential illness.

5. **Seek out social support.** Every year millions of people find themselves between cancer and good health, between a new lease on life and a new life of painful and life-changing medical treatment. Recognize that you are not alone. Open up to your family members, your friends, and your community. Accept their support. Find an advocate if you are able, and take advantage of the useful resources on the Internet and in the cancer community.

After weeks of uncertainty, John almost felt a sense of relief when his oncologist told him that he had cancer. Now he could finally move to the next stage. He could take action. He could deal with the situation. But he could not move on alone. John talked to Beth and his two closest friends. He shared his worries. He began to research his illness. Most days, he managed to walk or bike. These activities helped him make it through the beginning of his ordeal. They helped to make his new worrisome existential uncertainty a little bit easier to bear.

2 SOUNDING OFF ABOUT ULTRASOUND

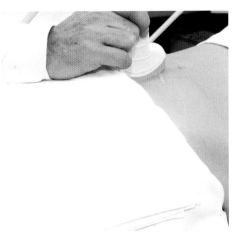

Once John's doctor had found the mass in his stomach, his path to diagnosis began. He had never had an ultrasound, so he read about the experience. "An ultrasound scan uses high frequency sound waves to create an image of part of the body continued with ultrasound." Ultrasounds are said to be safe (http://www.medicalnewstoday.com/articles/245491.php).

John learned that the test was safe, which reduced his anxiety somewhat. He knew he would be asked to remove his shirt and have cold jelly spread over his abdomen. On his way to the radiology department at his local hospital, he didn't spend much time pondering the ins and outs of the procedure. Instead, he wondered about the test results. What would they indicate? What would follow?

Ruminating about these troubling thoughts, John entered the radiology department and announced the time for his appointment. The admitting nurse gave him various forms to fill out and asked for his medical insurance card. When he turned the forms in, she asked him to sit in the waiting room until someone called his name. He sat among strangers who, from the diversity of their dress and subjects of conversation, hailed from all walks of life, representing all the social classes. All of them had come into this room with a range of concerns. He wondered what had brought the other patients to radiology—a broken bone, a mammogram, a sonogram, or perhaps a case similar to his mysterious abdominal mass. As he waited, the numbing sound of daytime television—talk shows—filled the air.

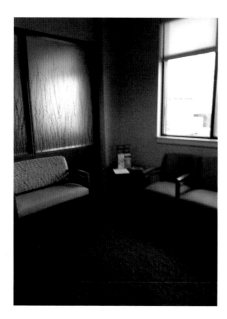

Trying to take his mind off his suddenly murky future, John looked at the magazines that had been placed on the table—People, US Weekly, Field & Stream, an old issue of Time, Vogue, and Ladies' Home Journal, as well as that day's edition of the local newspaper. In the absence of reading material, he scanned his phone for messages and e-mails, but even they could not ease his anxiety.

After what seemed an interminable stretch of time, a short woman dressed in green hospital scrubs called his name. He stood up. They introduced themselves.

The woman said in a cheerful tone:

"How are you today, John?"

"Just fine," John answered. John wondered if there was another possible answer to this question. What was he supposed to say? He wanted to tell her, "How do you think I am? I've been waiting for 30 minutes wondering if I'm going to live or die in the near future." But, of course, John, like most of us in that set of circumstances, remained silent.

"Follow me," the woman said, leading him into a windowless room with a couch, next to which was the ultrasound machine.

The woman asked him to remove his shirt and lie down on his back. John complied.

"Just so you know," the woman said, "this jelly is going to be cold as I spread it across your abdomen."

She turned on the machine and placed the ultrasound wand over John's stomach, moving it slowly in circles. At times she stopped the wand and pressed it on a particular spot. From his position, John watched her as she looked at the screen, wondering what she was seeing. On two occasions she asked him to shift his position. After about 30 minutes, she removed the water-based jelly and asked him to put on his shirt.

"Is that it?" he asked.

"Nothing to it," she said.

"How did it look?"

"Sorry, sir, I can't discuss the results. They have to be analyzed by a radiologist, who will send a report to your doctor."

"Can you give me any indication?"

"Sorry, sir," she said pleasantly. "Talk with your doctor."

As she shook John's hand, she said ominously, "I wish you the best of luck."

DEALING WITH DIAGNOSTIC STRESS

It is nearly impossible to be nonchalant about one's experience in the radiology department. It is, after all, a stressful place. Consider the elements that are combined to create this stressful environment. We are in a strange setting, a waiting room, full of strangers who are either reading, sitting nervously, or watching daytime television. The anxiety of others in the room is evident. We are welcomed by support staff who are clearly overworked, filling out paperwork, scanning the computer for insurance confirmations, and printing out prescriptions and procedure orders. It is not easy to interact with patients who are themselves worried about their future.

The technicians are trained to be polite and friendly, but how many ultrasound procedures will they perform in one morning? To make matters worse, patients never see the radiologists who spend their time hidden away in rooms in which they look at an endless stream of sonograms, X-rays, MRIs, and CT scans, making highly informed, life-changing judgments about what they see.

At the time of an ultrasound, the patient doesn't see what the technician or, ultimately, the radiologist will see. After the procedure, the technician says goodbye, and the patient has to wait several days for radiological analysis, which is then sent to the primary care physician, who, at an appointed time, will discuss the results of the procedure and recommend a course of action.

In cases like John's—potential cancer cases—the ultrasound procedure is used to see if cancer can be ruled out. It is a first step in the diagnostic process. If it reveals nothing of concern, which can be the case, then the patient can move on with her or his life. Invariably patients have to wait several excruciatingly stressful days to hear about the results.

In short, there is nothing one can do to avoid the existential elements that trigger stress in potential cancer patients. But we think there are a number of things we can do to make the ultrasound experience a bit more tolerable. In John's case, the ultrasound was the first step in a series of unpleasant and stressful situations. In order to avoid ruminating about the results of the test, John went home, drank a glass of wine, chatted with Beth, and decided to watch the most gripping film he could find. He wanted to take his mind off of his stressful day. He had a feeling there would be more stressful days to come.

SUGGESTIONS FOR CONFRONTING THE ULTRASOUND EXPERIENCE

1. **Rely on your social support.** There is no reason to confront an ultrasound procedure completely alone. Go with a friend or family member, preferably one who likes conversation, which makes waiting for the test easier to bear.
1. **Bring your favorite music.** In the absence of conversation, bring a device with earphones and listen to your favorite music.
1. **If possible, choose your facility.** There are some imaging centers that share preliminary results. Find one of these, if possible, to avoid having to wait for results.

3 THE INS AND OUTS OF CT SCANS

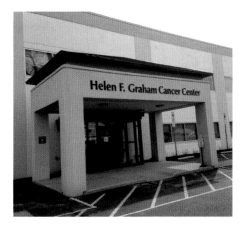

One of the most stressful times for anyone concerned about a potential illness is the waiting period between diagnostic procedures and the results of those tests. John was no exception. Anxious to find out the results of his ultrasound, he made an appointment with his primary care physician as soon as possible. Not wanting to discuss the possibilities he faced until he had more information, he kept his appointment to himself and went to the appointment alone.

John's stoicism did not blunt his anxiety, which had slowly increased day by day. When he entered his doctor's office, it reached a crescendo. In the past he had always felt comfortable in this space—small waiting room, a paper processing office with files, computers and phones that gave way to a narrow corridor that led to four examination rooms. The doctor's office was at the back of the space. John said hello to the office staff. The three women, all of whom had known him for more than 10 years, greeted him cheerfully, and led him immediately to the first examination room on the left, a square space with a desk, a blood pressure device, various medical tools and supplies, an examination table and several chairs. Most doctors' offices seemed to look identical. John wondered if they had conducted research that had somehow determined that a "sterile" and "cheerless" setting was the best way to "comfort" patients. His heart pounding, John sat down and tried read a magazine. He flipped through the pages absentmindedly, not reading anything. Finally his doctor, Peter, knocked on the door.

Like John, Peter was tall and thin and had a reassuring manner. John had known him for more than 15 years and trusted his judgment. After greeting John, Peter immediately began discussing the results of the test.

"They found something there. It's big, and unfortunately we don't know what it is."

John felt his world tilt slightly. The words were painful to hear. He didn't know how to reply. His worst fears might have come true.

"It could be nothing. We need to do more tests to rule out possibilities," Peter said calmly. His steady manner quieted John's nerves slightly.

"Possibilities?" John repeated.

Neither one of them wanted to say the word "cancer." John suddenly realized why people sometimes either whispered the word or did all they could to avoid saying it.

"We should schedule a CT scan for a better look at the mass. That will give us a better idea of what's going on," Peter continued.

John said nothing.

"It's probably nothing, John. You're in good physical shape. You shouldn't worry too much. We'll schedule the CT scan for you."

"Thank you," John said quietly.

Shaken, John left the examination room and stopped at the office. He presented his insurance card. Even in the midst of all his anxiety, John was grateful he had good insurance. At least the cost of these diagnostic tests would not be another item on his growing list of worries. He knew that many people did not have good insurance.

The receptionist gave him a CT scan order and arranged the date for the procedure. She also gave him a card with another doctor's name on it—a specialist in medical oncology. John would always remember that moment when he took his first steps into the world of cancer. His path had just taken a very unexpected and unpleasant turn.

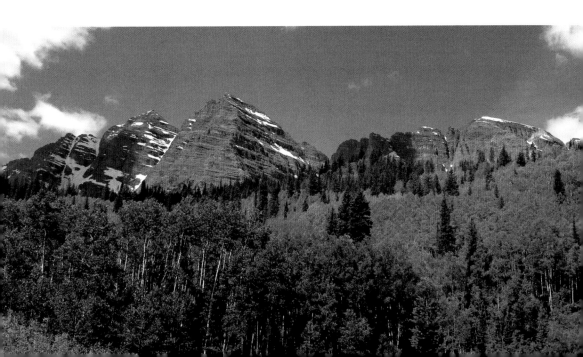

A WAY FORWARD

Initial encounters in the world of cancer are frightening. No one should have to face them alone. John realized that in the future he would ask Beth or one of his close friends to go with him to these appointments. It would be good to have someone hold his hand. Although John's experience would have been no less traumatic, it probably would have been a bit easier to bear if his wife, Beth, or his brother, Sean, or his best friend and law partner, Daniel, had been there with him. They might have held his hand, put an arm around his shoulder, patted him on the back, or told him that things will work out. Instead, John had mistakenly thought it would be easier to go alone, hear the results, and move on. Having thought of himself as a stoic male, he had now been forced to confront the first step up the mountain by himself. How frightening to walk and find the ground crumbling away.

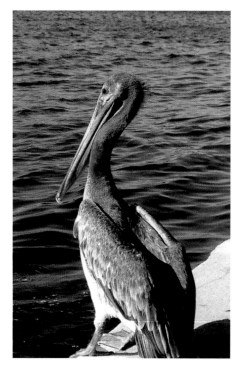

Everyone needs help to cope with an illness, especially one as potentially devastating as cancer. John realized that he needed to put aside his longstanding view of himself as an independent and strong person. This realization is one that most patients face at some point along their path. Our social expectations often encourage independence. Relying on someone is sometimes seen as weak. John decided he would never again be reluctant to ask someone for help. He was lucky to have reached this conclusion very early on in his illness. From now on, he would seek the help of his family and friends as he proceeded along the diagnostic path and beyond.

THE CT SCAN PROCEDURE

John, of course, still didn't know exactly what was going on. No one wanted to or was able to speculate about what they suspected: that John had a malignant tumor growing in his body. His brief experience with the first stage of the diagnostic process had already shaken him. He knew he needed to brace himself for the next stage. To get through the CT scan, he asked Beth to go with him.

A CT or CAT scan is a type of X-ray test that produces cross-sectional images of the body using X-rays and a computer. It is used for diagnosing medical diseases. The founders of this important procedure, Hounsfield and Cormack, were jointly awarded the Nobel Prize in 1979. A CT scan can help doctors to visualize small nodules or tumors, which they cannot see with a plain film X-ray.

http://www.emedicinehealth.com/ct_scan/article_em.htm

Beth helped John to prepare for the procedure. She made sure that he fasted the morning of his appointment and that he managed to drink the requisite bottles of unpleasant barium solution, which increased the contrast of the CT image. Such contrast would ensure a more accurate diagnosis. Beth also reminded John to wear loose-fitting clothing that had no metal, which would alter the images. John was grateful for her help and support. His anxiety made it difficult to remember details. Wanting to get the procedure over with as soon as possible, John had requested the first appointment of the day.

Beth drove to the hospital. During the drive, John silently prayed that the CT scan would be normal. He would be so grateful for a normal result, which would enable him to happily resume his life. In that moment all of his previous worries seemed inconsequential. "You never know what it could show," Beth said as they walked into the hospital and found their way to the radiology department. They checked in, settled into the waiting area, and flipped through magazines. John briefly wondered if anyone in any waiting room had ever actually read one of those magazines. Thankfully, the wait was short. A nurse called John's name and asked him to follow her into a wide hallway that gave way to a series of rooms that housed the imaging machines. She greeted him briefly and asked him to sit on a chair. She then looked at a list and began to ask a series of questions.

"Did you drink your barium?" she asked him.

"Yes."

"Good, have a bit more," she said giving him a small cupful. "It will help with the results."

"Did you fast?"

"Yes."

"I see you dressed appropriately—no metal."

"Is someone here with you?" she asked.

John nodded.

"Do you mind if we start the IV now? Right or left arm?"

"Left." John rolled up his loose shirt and held out his arm.

The nurse mentioned that John had good veins. "It looks like you work out."

"I bike, play golf, and try to work out at the gym." John mumbled his answers, trying not to think about golf or the gym.

The nurse nodded. "You're not allergic to latex or iodine, are you?"

"Not that I know about," John answered nervously.

"Good" She expertly put the IV in on the underside of his elbow and then led him to

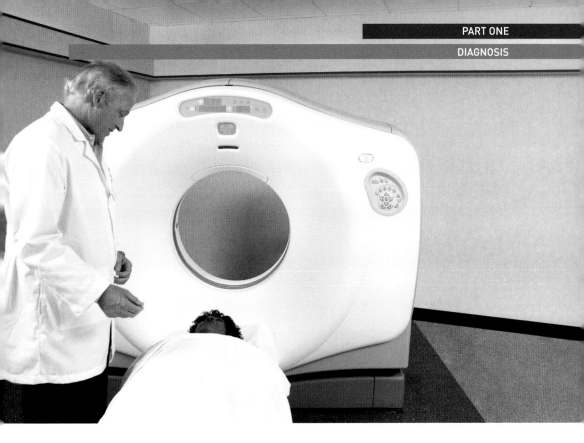

the CT room, a large space kept quite cool for an optimum operating environment.

There the nurse introduced him to the CT technician, who noticed John staring at the CT machine, a big, round, gleaming, and somewhat frightening instrument.

"They're much better than they used to be," the technician said cheerfully as the nurse left. "It used to take 45 minutes to get the images, but now it's much quicker." She asked John to lie down on the gurney and gave him a bolster to put under this knees and a blanket to keep him warm. She asked him to put his arms over his head. "Just follow the verbal instructions about holding your breath. We'll take two sets of images—one without contrast, and one with."

She attached John's IV to the container near the machine that held iodine contrast. "When the first set of images is done, you'll feel the iodine—warmth spreading through your arms, chest, and pelvis. You might get a metallic taste on the roof of your mouth. Don't worry, that's normal."

"Normal?"

"Ready?"

John nodded.

"Okay, I'm going to run things from the room behind the protective glass."

"Because of radiation?" John asked.

"That's right, but it's still safe for you," she said reassuringly as she left the room. The machine began to whir. The gurney moved John into a variety of positions under the scanner. When instructed, John held his breath. Lying on the gurney, he wondered what the images looked like. He tried to think pleasant thoughts—a walk or bike ride—but the constant instruction made it difficult. After about 20 minutes, the technician came back into the room.

"You did great." She asked him to sit up slowly. Then she removed his IV, and put a bandage on his arm.

"How did it look?" John asked.

"I don't know. The radiologist will review the images, draft a report, and send it on to your doctor. Good luck," she added, which sounded ominous to John. As quickly as his shaky legs would take him, John dressed and found Beth. They left the hospital. Since John had been fasting, Beth suggested they stop for an early lunch. He felt grateful for her company. They found a local diner and had some excellent omelets and toast. For John, each of these "normal" activities now seemed to hold a special significance.

THE RISKS AND BENEFITS OF CT SCANS

Patients should know the risks and benefits of CT scans. CT scans enable professionals to pinpoint and stage tumors. They aid in diagnosis and enable oncologists to track the progress of therapies. By the same token, CT scans expose patients to radiation, which can have negative effects. Too much radiation increases the risk of developing a secondary cancer. Patients undergoing a series of CT scans should be aware of these risks and benefits.

ADDITIONAL INFORMATION ON CT SCANS AND RADIATION

1. How Much Do CT Scans Increase the Risk of Cancer? Researchers reevaluate the safety of radiation used in medical imaging. Jun 18, 2013 |By Carina Storrs Scientific American http://www. scientificamerican.com/article/how-much-ct-scans-increase-risk-cancer/.

2. American College of Radiology. Patient Safety: Radiation Dose in X-rays and CT Scans. http://www.radiologyinfo.org/en/safety/?pg=sfty_xray.

3. US Food and Drug Administration. Computed Tomography. http://www.fda.gov/RadiationEmittingProducts/ RadiationEmittingProductsandProcedures/MedicalImaging/ MedicalX-Rays/ucm115317.htm.

4. The American Cancer Society. General Comments and Questions on Radiation Risk. http://www.fda.gov/Radiation-EmittingProducts/ RadiationEmittingProductsandProcedures/MedicalImaging/ MedicalX-Rays/ucm115317.htm

5. The most common procedures for cancer diagnosis are described at the website below: http://www.cancer.net/navigating-cancer-care/ diagnosing-cancer/tests-and-procedures

WAITING FOR DIAGNOSTIC RESULTS

Waiting for diagnostic results is not unlike a defendant waiting for a jury's verdict. During that period of time, the defendant wonders if he or she will be sentenced to death, to years in jail, probation, community service or, better yet, set free. The same can be said of the wait for the results of diagnostic procedures. How will the findings change one's life, if at all?

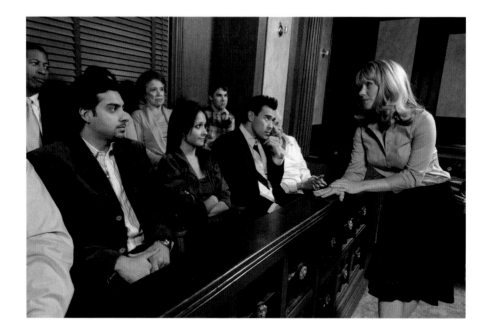

There is no easy way for anyone to get through this difficult period. Like John, people sometimes bury themselves in the details of their work. Some people may take a short trip or reduce their anxiety by drinking alcohol or smoking marijuana. Still other people will simply deny that a problem exists, moving on with their everyday lives as if nothing had changed. Some people might pass the time through meditation, increased exercise, or prayer in a church, synagogue, or a mosque. But no matter what we do, the specter of an uncertain future remains and will continue to be present until there is a definitive diagnosis, which, given the complexities of cancer, can sometimes take weeks or months.

In this regard John was lucky; it took just a few days for the results to come in. Accompanied by Beth, he went to his appointment. As they located the oncologist's office and walked up a flight of stairs, John gazed at a large sign that read Cancer Center. He was amazed at how quickly his life had turned upside down. He had never talked with an oncologist before—he had never had the need to do so. The oncologist was a pleasant-looking, middle-aged man who was short and fit. He smiled warmly at John and Beth and introduced himself as Fred. He greeted John and Beth and asked John to come back to an examination room.

There, he took John's medical history and did a routine physical, checking his reflexes. He palpated his abdomen.

"I can feel it," he said as he pressed on the spot where the tumor had grown. "Let's go talk in the office."

He led John back to his office and asked Beth to join them. Behind his desk, John's CT scans were illuminated on the screen, and for the first time, John saw his tumor, a swirling mass that looked like a bank of storm clouds in the black expanse of his abdomen. The doctor said that the tumor looked as if it had been growing for some time. It was the size of a small grapefruit. The doctor was not certain if it was malignant.

"Not all tumors are malignant. This one, which is wrapped around your aorta, is a pretty good size, but it could be benign. We need to do a biopsy to see what kind of cells make up the tumor."

"Can you cut it out?" Beth asked.

"Probably not," Fred said. "If it is malignant, we'll have to use chemotherapy drugs to reduce and hopefully eliminate the tumor."

John shuddered. He once again quickly wondered how he could have cancer when he felt so well. He had done all the "right things." He followed a healthy diet, he exercised, and he had a positive attitude about his life. He had a good life. He liked his work, and he had supportive colleagues and a loving wife. How could he get cancer?

John and Beth had thought that this meeting would resolve the indeterminacies of diagnosis. But like many other cancer patients, John's diagnostic journey was not yet over. John needed a biopsy. Most biopsies are rather routine procedures, but John's would take place in his abdomen, a crowded place where indiscriminate probing could pierce his intestine. So the oncologist ordered a biopsy guided by CT images—much more complicated. This procedure required another CT scan during which a biopsy would be performed. Once again accompanied by Beth,

John made his way to the now-familiar hospital and placed himself in the hands of nurses and technicians. He hoped that they all knew what they were doing, but he was already beginning to feel somewhat helpless about the unexpected and unpleasant route his life had taken.

The procedure took several hours. When it was finally over, he found Beth in the waiting room. This time neither of them suggested stopping for food. They just wanted to get home. They knew that they would, once again, have the anxiety of yet another period of waiting—for results, for the verdict that would determine John's future.

Even though John had Beth and his family and friends, all of whom were concerned about John's future and who phoned or visited him throughout this process, John felt very much alone. He appreciated their support, but at this juncture their words of encouragement did not calm him. He was very afraid—for his life. Confronted by a looming and treacherous mountain, he didn't know what to do.

PATIENT ADVOCACY

When people find themselves in John's situation, it is very difficult to make the decisions—fateful decisions—that the medical establishment compels us to make. Some people are able to find comfort in a patient advocate—someone who knows the ins and outs of medical insurance, diagnostic innovations, new treatments, and impressive clinical trials. The advocate is a professional at the cutting edge of medical practice. The right advocate can help us make informed and rational decisions for our particular set of medical circumstances.

Patient advocates represent a patient when he or she is in need of medical care. They help the patient through a difficult time and a complicated decision-making process. Like John, most patients are confused and may feel helpless in the face of medical tests, diagnosis, and treatment decisions. A patient advocate can guide patients through this maze, offering advice. They simplify, explain, and help patients get the best possible care. Advocates can be found in a variety of places, such as hospitals and non-profit agencies (http://www.assertivepatient.

org/patient-advocate.html). Luckily for John, he had an old college friend who was a patient advocate.

When John and Beth got home from the biopsy procedure, John decided he would call Daniel and ask if he could take him on as a patient. The decision made him feel a bit less helpless.

RESOURCES FOR PATIENT ADVOCACY

1. Patient Advocate Foundation: help@patientadvocate.org. Phone: (800) 532-5274; Fax: (757) 873-8999.
2. National Patient Safety Foundation: 268 Summer Street · 6th Floor Boston, MA 02210 USA www. npsf.org.
3. ADVO Connection Directory: www.advoconnection.com

THE BIOPSY

It had now been roughly one month since John had first gone to see his doctor for a "check-up." It had been a month filled with anxiety, a month during which his life had changed dramatically. Compared to the looming mountain that he now faced, his previous worries and concerns now seemed insignificant.

John still did not know if he had cancer. If he did have it, he didn't know what kind it might be. Worse yet, he would have to undergo more tests to achieve a definitive diagnosis and learn about his prognosis. Based on the cellular analysis of the tumor tissue, Fred could determine if the cells were indeed malignant, and then determine, if necessary, the kind and grade of the potentially malignant cancer cells.

When John and Beth returned to see the oncologist, they had already prepared themselves for the worst. Even so, John held out hope that his tumor was benign. They all sat down and unsuccessfully attempted to make small talk. Fred took a deep breath and told John that he had cancer.

"You have a low grade follicular lymphoma," he told them. "You should know that the treatment for this kind of cancer is quite effective," he added quickly, knowing how the news would affect John.

There were a few moments of tense silence, during which time neither Beth nor John could think of a single question to pose. Finally Fred gave them some pamphlets about treatment options. He briefly summarized them. He asked John to talk with his advocate and friend, Daniel. He suggested that they take two weeks and then return with a treatment decision. In the interim, Fred would be available to talk about any issues John might have. John very much appreciated Fred's straightforward and calm manner.

Fred also recommended yet one more procedure: a bone marrow biopsy, which would be performed in-house.

"When could that be done?" John asked. He was already preparing to proceed to the next stage of his experience.

"Right now. We can do it in the office. It is painful but lasts only a moment. In the long run it is less stressful than going back to the hospital."

After some preparation, Fred used a needle to remove a sample of John's bone marrow to check to see if lymphoma cells had spread there. The procedure turned out to be very painful. John was glad he had gotten it over with. At least he didn't have to worry about going to the hospital for yet another procedure.

John had never experienced such a day. First, he learned that he had cancer. Second, he had to undergo an unexpected and painful bone marrow biopsy. John and Beth finally returned home in a state of shock. Although only three hours had transpired, it seemed like a lifetime.

When John got home, he went online to read up on NHL, a set of cancers of which none, he learned, are officially curable. "These are cancers that can be 'managed' but not 'cured,'" he told Beth after an hour of reading.

"I'll try to get the best care I can get," John told Beth, once again attempting to be the stoic. He added: "I will get through this. You'll see."

"I know you'll be okay, John. Let's try not to let this control our whole life," Beth said. She had also been conducting research online about how to cope with cancer. Evidently much of her research had indicated it would be helpful to continue with "life as usual." Beth had decided that she would help John through her calm approach to cancer. She would encourage him to continue his activities (as much as possible) and make sure that he saw his friends and family regularly.

"We have to go on as before," she told him. "That means that you should try to continue to work and exercise as much as possible."

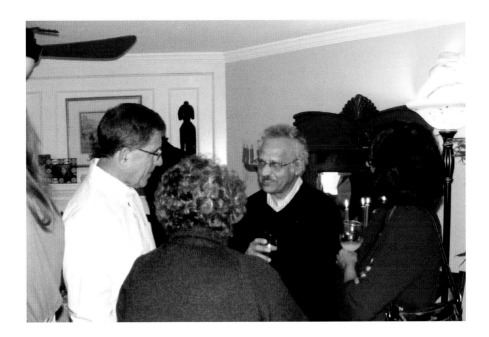

LETTING PEOPLE KNOW

John and Beth now faced the daunting task of telling their friends and family that John did, in fact, have cancer. How do we tell our loved ones that we have a serious disease like cancer? What could be more difficult? How do we tell them that our cancer has no cure? John and Beth were overwhelmed. They wondered how their friends would react. They knew that people would be sad, concerned, and perhaps uncomfortable. In the past, John had never seemed to know what to say to people who had shared bad news with him. He decided that the best course of action was to be direct. Not wanting to be stoic again, he wanted to admit his fear, but also tell people that he was coping with this life transition. He wanted to tell his friends that he wanted to continue to lead an active life as much as possible. He did not want all of his conversations to be about cancer. He knew that he had good people in his life and that they would be supportive. This realization made the entire situation easier to bear.

There is no easy solution to the many challenges that cancer presents. One way to feel less isolated in the world is to read or watch cancer testimonials. They can be easily found within cancer discussion groups affiliated with the major cancer organizations, like the American Cancer Society, or the websites of major hospitals, like Memorial Sloan Kettering Cancer Center or the Fox Chase Cancer, to name two of several that are National Cancer Institute Centers of Comprehensive Cancer Care. There are also a wide variety of cancer memoirs that are in wide circulation. These cancer stories do not alleviate our concerns, but they can suggest ways to cope with personal and familial stresses and strains. They may provide a glimmer of hope in dire circumstances.

John and Beth shared John's news with their friends and family. It was less stressful than anticipated. Several of their friends made suggestions and provided advice. Although such unsolicited advice was not what they wanted to hear, they appreciated the effort and concerns of their friends. They were grateful to have a network of support. They were glad they had a patient advocate to guide them through the medical maze. They appreciated the fact that they could make choices about care without worrying about the costs.

Beth decided to read the memoirs of cancer patients in order to more fully understand how John might be feeling. There are, of course, many cancer memoirs to consider. There are memoirs written from a male perspective, from a woman's point of view, from a physician's orientation, or from a writer's experience.

There are scientific books that take spiritual, personal, or cultural perspectives. Thankfully, there is help for those who are seeking it. In this literature there are messages of hope and testaments of forbearance as well as tales of coping with pain and anxiety. All of them can help patients to cope with the uncertainties and stresses of learning that they have cancer.

CANCER MEMOIRS TO CONSIDER

1. Broyard, Anatol, Aleandra (Compiler). 1993. *Intoxicated by My Illness.* New Ballatine Books.
2. Bishop, Bryan. 2014. *Manhood, Marriage, and the Tumor That Tried to Kill Me.* New York: Thomas Dunn Books.
3. Carr, Kate. 2005. *It's Not Like That, Actually: A Memoir of Surviving Cancer – And Beyond.* New York: Vermillion.
4. Drescher, Fran. 2005. *Cancer Schmancer.* New York: Warner Books.
5. Rogers, Joni. 2002. *Bald in the Land of Big Hair: A True Story.* New York: Harper Perennial.

PERSONAL EXPERIENCE AND TREATMENT CHOICE

The experience of other cancer patients, however helpful, is no substitute for one's own experience. Another person's story can be revelatory, but it can never substitute for our own story. Another person's story may give us comfort and make us feel less lonely in the world, but it usually cannot solve all of our problems or make the challenges of confronting cancer disappear into the mists above the mountain.

John and Beth read several cancer memoirs and watched several cancer videos. In the end, though, they realized that John had to make his own way up the mountain. He had to choose the ascent best suited to his needs. The first challenge, of course, was to make a treatment decision. In cancer, these decisions are not always clear-cut. The oncologist presented John with three options: watch and wait; traditional chemotherapy; and chemotherapy combined with the more aggressive approach of immunotherapy. Because John had not experienced the symptoms of his slow-growing disease, he could simply postpone treatment until symptoms eventually developed.

John also had the choice of beginning treatment with standard chemotherapy, which has a track record of bringing lymphoma patients into remissions of varying lengths. Finally, he could elect a more aggressive immunotherapeutic treatment that had shown great promise in providing remissions of much longer duration.

After considerable thought and discussion, John decided on the more aggressive therapy. It seemed right for him, but such a decision might not be a good one for other patients. As we stated previously, to make the most informed decisions, it is, at times, helpful to employ a patient advocate. John and Beth both found Daniel's support to be extremely helpful. If an advocate is too costly, information about treatment options is provided and discussed on various websites. For each kind of cancer, there are websites that provide an array of information and perspectives on treatment options. Here are a few of them.

Treatment Options on Cancer Websites

1. For all kinds of cancers, consult the National Cancer Institute: http://www.cancer.gov.
2. For blood cancers, connect to the Leukemia and Lymphoma Society: http://www.lls.org/diseaseinformation/lymphoma/nonhodgkinlymphoma/
3. For lung cancer, consult the Lung Cancer Alliance: http://www.lungcanceralliance.org/
4. For breast cancer, link up with the National Breast Cancer Foundation, Inc.: http://www.lungcanceralliance.org/.
5. For colorectal cancer, consider the Colon Cancer Alliance: http://www.lungcanceralliance.org

Each kind of cancer also has allied organizations and hospital centers that provide a wealth of information about each specific kind of disease. The sheer magnitude of information, however, can sometimes make the treatment decision-making process extremely difficult. Given a seemingly endless array of possibilities, each one having its positive and negative aspects, how do we decide on a course of action? Because John led an active life, he believed that he was strong enough to withstand the most aggressive treatment, one that held the promise, though not the certainty, of a long remission.

4 DOCTOR–PATIENT RELATIONS

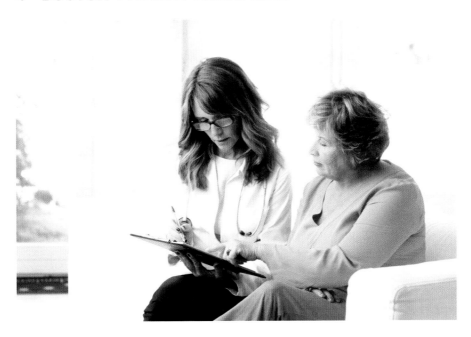

One of the most important aspects of any treatment regime is the patient–doctor relationship. This is especially true in the case of serious illnesses such as cancer. It is unfortunate that this relationship is often not as satisfying as it could be. In fact, studies have shown that many people are dissatisfied with the medical system, especially with their physicians. All too often they feel rushed in and out of consultations. They feel that their needs are not sufficiently heard.

The corporatization of medicine is certainly one cause of this dissatisfaction. Doubts about the quality of one's medical care are another reason for concern.

Surveys suggest that medical care in the United States is no longer considered the "best in the world." In a January 14, 2010, editorial calling for American health care reform, the *New England Journal of Medicine* cited a 2000 World Health Organization (WHO) survey that ranked the U.S. health care system 37th in the world. Without a subsequent WHO survey, one cannot say for sure, but it is probable that the U.S. ranking has not improved. The whys and wherefores of contemporary medicine are daunting—both for physicians and for patients.

Physicians tend to be overworked. Given the constraints of the corporatized medical system, complex medical insurance regimens, and the legions of people who lack insurance, it's surprising that anyone can get decent medical treatment. There is increasingly less time for doctors to listen to their patients, let alone treat them as complex human beings who are in pain or concerned about their well-being. Consider the experience of Joan Eisenstodt, as reported by Roni Caryn Rabin in *Kaiser Heath News*.

> Joan Eisenstodt didn't have a stopwatch when she went to see an ear-nose-and-throat specialist recently, but she is certain the physician was not in the exam room with her for more than three or four minutes.

> "He looked up my nose, said it was inflamed, told me to see the nurse for a prescription and was gone," said the 66-year-old Washington, D.C., consultant, who was suffering from an acute sinus infection.

> When she started protesting the doctor's choice of medication, "He just cut me off totally," she said. "I've never been in and out from a visit faster."

Rabin reports that it is common for physicians to limit visits to 15 minutes. She says that in some hospitals, visits are logged in for 11 minutes. New doctors, according to Pauline Chen's report in the May 30th, 2013 edition of *The New York Times,* are spending even less time with patients—eight minutes on average. To make matters even more frustrating, the average wait for a doctor's appointment has increased. Here are some of the findings of a survey released in 2014 by Merritt Hawkins, a national health care research and consulting firm.

1. The average appointment wait time to see a family physician ranged from a high of 66 days in Boston to a low of 5 days in Dallas.
2. The average appointment wait time to see an obstetrician/gynecologist ranged from a high of 46 days in Boston to a low of 10 days in Seattle.
3. The average appointment wait time to see a dermatologist ranged from a high of 72 days in Boston to a low of 16 days in Miami.
4. The average appointment wait time to see a cardiologist ranged from a high of 32 days in Washington, D.C. to a low of 11 days in Atlanta.
5. The average appointment wait time to see an orthopedic surgeon ranged from a high of 18 days in San Diego to a low of 5 days in Philadelphia, Minneapolis, and Houston.
6. The average cumulative wait times to see a cardiologist in all 15 markets was 16.8 days, up from 15.5 days in 2004.

Time is not the only enemy of good doctor–patient relations. Consider the digitalization of medical records. In the 3 to 15 minutes in the examination room, much time is spent with the physician seated in front of her or his computer, asking questions and entering new data, or perhaps looking at radiographic images, a scenario that makes any kind of eye-contact (a central element in interpersonal relations) more difficult. There are, of course, exceptions. Primary care physicians tend to spend more time with patients than do specialists like cardiologists, surgeons, or oncologists.

Like all professionals, physicians have their strengths and weaknesses. There are some who are more skilled or knowledgeable than others. Some are relaxed, friendly, and outgoing; others are more reserved. Some deal with the stress of caring for their patients better than others. Some are able to listen to patients, while others tend to dismiss patient concerns. Some physicians "tell it like it is; others are more diplomatic about reporting the results of medical testing. These interpersonal skills have been important in medical education. For more than a decade, medical schools have been increasing the required amount of training in doctor-patient communication (see http://enews.tufts.edu/stories/794/2003/10/09/MedCom/).

Given these real-world time constraints, how can physicians and patients forge relationships of mutual trust and respect?

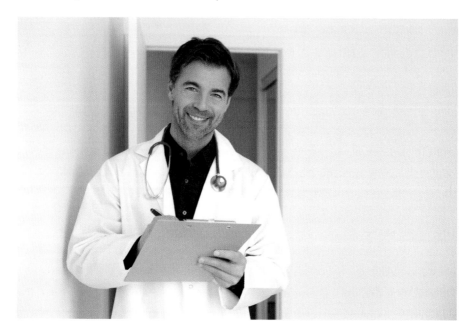

DOCTOR CONFIDENCE

John was fortunate. He liked his primary care physician, a man who was about his age and who had always taken the time to talk with him and explain things to him. He looked at John when they talked. He did not talk down to John. When recommending a medicine, he consulted John. In addition, John respected the fact that his physician was a deliberate and cautious doctor who did not believe in ordering unnecessary diagnostic tests. By the same token, he was a man who did not sugarcoat the results of tests. When he recommended an oncologist, he gave John the name of a physician who possessed professional qualities similar to his own.

"I think you will like him," he told John. "He's a straight shooter. If the prognosis is good, he'll tell you. If it's not, he will also tell what you can expect."

John trusted his doctor's judgment. He felt reassured when he met the man who would become his oncologist. The new oncologist, Fred, listened to his concerns, talked to him with respect, and answered his questions respectfully. Both John and Beth also felt that Fred possessed cutting-edge knowledge of oncological medicine. Although John's journey on the mountain trails of cancer would be fraught with peril, John felt that Fred would be a worthy guide who could hopefully help him find his way up the slope. Fred was also not adverse to complementary medicine. He talked respectfully about several possible options.

From the outset, Fred was interested in John's activities. He recommended that John walk, lift weights, and take up yoga. He asked questions about John's diet. He suggested John eat the foods he enjoyed and even drink a glass or two of wine.

This flexibility reinforced John's willingness to stay with this doctor. Having faith in his oncologist eased John's anxiety slightly. He was lucky that he did not have to interview doctor after doctor in an attempt to find one who was a good fit. In his present state, John was grateful for small blessings. Guided by an able oncologist, John moved forward to the next stage of his difficult journey up the mountain.

SUGGESTED RESOURCES ON DOCTOR–PATIENT RELATIONS

There is a large body of literature on doctor–patient relations. Below are just a few of these sources. Some of these are scholarly; others are more journalistic:

1. Ainsworth-Vaughn, Nancy. 1998. *Claiming Power in Doctor–Patient Talk*. New York: Oxford University Press.
2. Fisher, Sue and Alexandra Dundas Todd (eds.) *The Social Organization of Doctor–Patient Communication*. New York: Ablex
3. Fong Ha, Jennifer MBBS (Hons), Dip Surg Anat, and Nancy Longnecker, PhD. 2010. *Doctor–Patient Communication: A Review*. Ochsner Journal Spring 10(1): 38-43.
4. Gold, Susan Dorr, MD, MHSA, MA and Mack Lipkin, Jr., MD. 1999. *The Doctor–Patient Relationship: Challenges, Opportunities, and*

Strategies, Journal of General Internal Medicine (January) 14 (Suppl 1): S 26-33.

5. Rabin, Roni Caryn. 2014. 15-Minute Visits Take A Toll On The Doctor–Patient Relationship. *Kaiser Health News,* April 21, 2014.

6. The Daily Beast. *Is the Doctor–Patient Relationship Turning into a Business Partnership?* April 11, 2014.

5 ALTERNATIVE TREATMENTS

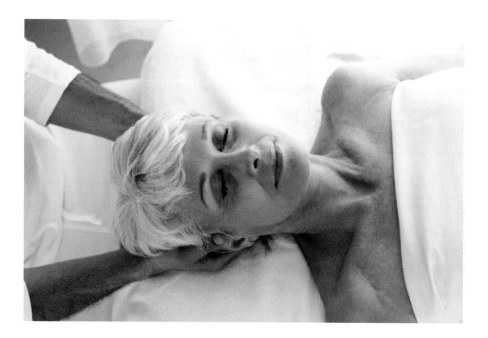

Establishing a satisfying rapport with our oncologists and making treatment choices are generally the first steps after diagnosis. Treatment for cancer often consists of combinations of chemotherapy and immunotherapy, radiation, or both. The start of this difficult ascent up the mountain is formidable. It is fraught with peril. Treatment regimens tend to produce harsh physical side effects—bone pain, mouth sores, loss of hair, loss of appetite, weight loss, fatigue, neuropathy, and anemia. They also carry with them psychological side effects, the most prominent of which are anxiety and clinical depression. If treatment is required to save our lives, an important question that accompanies that treatment is how do we best manage our treatment? What can we do to minimize the negative side effects? Are there ways to avoid losing our hair, to feel less anxious, and to maximize our energy levels?

Like other patients about to face cancer treatment, John pondered these questions. In some ways, John was once again lucky. Ten years prior to John's diagnosis, the negative effects of chemotherapy had been much worse. Considerable advances had been made in treatment since then, and survival rates had increased.

Some practitioners even developed strategies to prevent cancers altogether. Certain scientists, like Dr. Joseph Mercola, advocated special diets to prevent all cancers. They claimed that cancer cells thrive on sugar, which meant that if people reduced or eliminated sugar from their diets, cancer cells would not be able to reproduce. Although this path could be a possible preventative strategy, it's not at all scientifically clear if special diets can "cure" cancer. Here's what Dr. Mercola said about diet and treatment of cancers.

> Without a doubt the most powerful essential strategy I know of to treat cancer is to starve the cells by depriving them of their food source. Unlike your body cells, which can burn carbs or fat for fuel, cancer cells have lost that metabolic flexibility. Dr. Otto Warburg was actually given a Nobel Prize over 75 years ago for figuring this out, but virtually no oncologist actually uses this information.

> You can review my recent interview with Dr. D'Agostino below for more details, but integrating a ketogenic diet with hyperbaric oxygen therapy, which is deadly to cancer cells debilitated by starving them of their fuel source would be the strategy I would recommend to my family if they were diagnosed with cancer. (http://articles.mercola.com/sites/articles/archive/2013/08/03/natural-cancer-treatment.aspx)

There are more conventional approaches to alternative cancer treatments. Once a comprehensive evaluation has been conducted, a specialist might recommend a combination of treatments to supplement chemotherapy or radiation treatments.

In addition to their potential physical benefits, alternative treatments also tend to make patients like John feel that they are controlling aspects of their treatment and recovery. Alternative treatments also have the advantage of reducing the negative side effects of conventional treatments, such as nausea, pain, and anxiety. The Mayo clinic recommends 10 alternative treatment options. They have been shown to be beneficial and are safe to use. When considering an array of alternative therapies, it is important to work in consultation with a primary physician to coordinate these treatment methods.

If you're experiencing	Then consider trying
Anxiety	Hypnosis, massage, meditation, relaxation techniques
Fatigue	Exercise, massage, relaxation techniques, yoga
Nausea and vomiting	Acupuncture, aromatherapy, hypnosis, music therapy
Pain	Acupuncture, aromatherapy, hypnosis, massage, music therapy
Sleep problems	Exercise, relaxation techniques, yoga
Stress	Aromatherapy, exercise, hypnosis, massage, meditation, tai chi, yoga

http://www.mayoclinic.org/diseases-conditions/cancer/in-depth/cancer-treatment/art-20047246

ADDITIONAL SOURCES FOR ALTERNATIVE CANCER TREATMENTS

1. American Cancer Society: They provide information on herbs, oils, and minerals for alternative cancer treatment. http://www.cancer.org/treatment/treatmentsandsideeffects/complementaryandalternativemedicine/herbsvitaminsandminerals/index?sitearea=eto

2. The Cancer Tutor: The Future of Cancer Research http://www.cancertutor.com/

3. Hope 4 Cancer Institute: They provide information on alternative treatments. http://www.hope4cancer.com/treatments

4. The Gerson Institute: They provide information on nontoxic treatments for cancer. http://gerson.org/gerpress/

CHOOSING A SET OF ALTERNATIVE TREATMENTS

John's trust in his oncologist helped him decide on a treatment path. He would undergo chemotherapy for nine months. This daunting regimen would no doubt need to be supplemented with "alternative methods." John and Beth both believed in the power of age-old complementary treatment methods. They assumed that these methods would have long ago disappeared if they were not effective. Alternative treatment methods, or complementary and alternative medicine (CAM), can be defined as any healing approach that incorporates a holistic view of the person. These approaches, most of which have their origins in Eastern religious or philosophical traditions, have recently become very popular in the West.

There are a number of categories of complementary or alternative medicine. The National Center of Complementary and Alternative Medicine (NCCAM) recognizes five main categories. These include:

Mind–body medicine. Mind–body medicine includes treatments that focus on how our mental and emotional status interacts with and affects the body's ability to function. Examples include meditation and various therapies expressed through art and music.

Whole medical systems. This category refers to complete systems of medical theory and practice, many of which go back thousands of years and have roots in non-Western cultures. Examples include traditional Chinese medicine and Ayurveda, a therapy that originated in India. Whole medical systems from the West include homeopathy and naturopathy.

Manipulative and body-based practices. Relying on physical manipulation of the body, this practice is intended to improve specific symptoms and overall health. Examples of these practices include chiropractic and osteopathy.

Energy medicine. This form of alternative medicine uses energy fields to promote healing. Biofield therapies that affect the energy fields that are said to encircle the human body include Reiki and qi gong. Bioelectromagnetic-based treatments, such as magnet therapy, involve the manipulation of electromagnetic fields.

Biologically based practices. Here the focus is on herbs, nutrition, and vitamins, dietary supplements, and herbal medicine. They constitute the most common forms of biologically based complementary and alternative medicine. A growing interest in these kinds of therapies has prompted more research about their effectiveness. Even so, many of these biologically based practices have yet to be thoroughly tested.

http://www.everydayhealth.com/alternative-health/the-basics.aspx

Studies have found that between 30 and 40 percent of Americans tend to rely on some form of complementary or alternative medicine. Those who embrace these treatment procedures, like Beth and John, tend to be highly educated and able to conduct research on the benefits and drawbacks of various treatment measures. Like many other Americans, John and Beth embraced the notion of integrative medicine, an approach in which practitioners combine traditional and contemporary medical orientations to healing.

John was especially pleased to learn that CAM practitioners focus on the entire person, incorporating a mind–body approach to the person. Since finding out about his tumor, John had been feeling somewhat disconnected from his body. The more he learned about CAM treatments, the more he liked the holistic philosophy of these treatment options.

Once a treatment decision had been made, John and Beth discussed possible alternative treatments. Their research yielded a wide range of choices, making it difficult to understand all of the possibilities. They wondered if these "natural alternative therapies" really reduced the toxic side effects of chemotherapy, radiation, and, to a lesser extent, immunotherapy. They were both very concerned about John's ability to tolerate the difficult treatment ahead. Their patient advocate helped them gain a clearer picture of the vast alternative therapy landscape. Their advocate informed them of results from new research clinical trials, which, in turn, eased the burden of John's decision-making.

John would soon undergo traditional chemotherapy mixed with protocols of immunotherapy. It would be painful and difficult, but he and Beth felt confident that

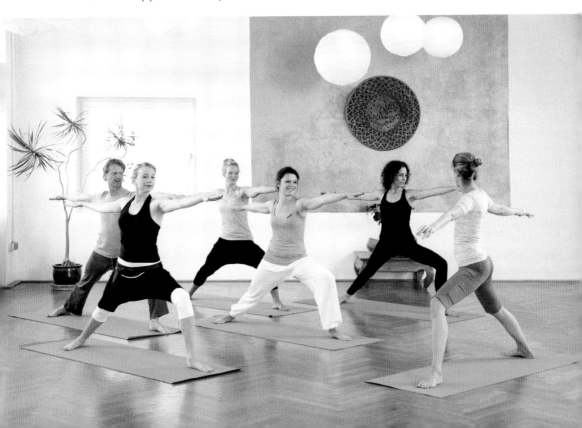

this path was the right one for John to follow. The combination of chemotherapy and immunotherapy (which uses the body's immune system to destroy cancer cells) would be John's best course of action. Given the expected side effects, they looked into courses of action that would reduce their intensity.

THE BENEFITS OF EXERCISE

John had a lifelong belief in the benefits of physical activity. He had always been active. As a child he played sports. As an adult he biked, ran, hiked, and played golf. As he read about how to promote healing from cancer, John found a large body of research that advocated physical activity. John and Beth also read the testimonials of cancer patients who claimed physical fitness was one of the best defenses against the ravages of chemotherapy.

In fact, physical activity has long been linked to the promotion of good health. Such activity appears to be beneficial whether we are struggling with a chronic illness like John or simply trying to maintain a state of good health. Regular physical activity can control weight, reduce the risk of heart disease, reduce the risk of diabetes, prevent or reduce the risk of cancers, strengthen the body, promote immune system health, improve mood, and reduce anxiety (http://www.cdc.gov/physicalactivity/everyone/health/index.html?s_cid=cs_284).

If practiced properly, there appear to be very few negative ramifications associated with physical activity. Unlike John, the majority of Americans do not engage in physical activity. It is important for anyone who wants to become active to start slowly and discuss their plans with their physician. As for John, he hoped that his high degree of fitness would help him to withstand the hardships associated with chemo. He hoped that he would be able to remain active. Studies support John's belief that exercise might increase his vitality during chemotherapy.

One study reported in the *British Medical Journal* by L. Adamsen in October, 2009, examined the effect of different intensity exercises on chemotherapy patients. Two hundred and sixty-nine cancer patients representing 21 different types of cancer participated in the study. They were required to take part in a six-week program that included high intensity cardiovascular exercise, resistance training, relaxation, and body awareness training and massage therapy. At the end of the study, researchers found a marked decrease in tiredness, and improved vitality, muscle strength, aerobic capacity, and physical activity (http://www.livestrong.com/article/395995-exercise-during-chemotherapy/).

Beth had always encouraged John to maintain his fitness routine, and now was no exception. John committed to maintaining as much of his exercise regime as possible. He also realized that an activity routine would give him a sense of normality. He realized that he would have to alter his normal activities but would do what he could.

After considerable research John and Beth came to several conclusions about alternative therapies. Beth recommended that John begin to reduce his sugar intake and take a vitamin D supplement daily.

"And," she added, "we should try to take some yoga and meditation classes. Who knows, maybe we will like it."

"I've never been a yoga person," John said, "and you know it's hard for me to sit still for more than a moment. I wonder if I can learn to meditate?"

"You never know," Beth said. "Who would have thought you would be facing a serious illness? One thing is for certain; life is full of unexpected twists and turns— some good ones, and bad ones. No matter what, our life is going to change."

"I like having my feet massaged," John said, "so maybe I can start with reflexology. I've read that reflexology is good for the side effects of chemotherapy."

John was embarking on a variety of new treatment procedures, some by necessity, others by choice. John hoped to find his way through an unexpectedly dense and confusing situation.

PRELUDE TO TREATMENT

In the coming chapters, we discuss John's difficult climb up the mountain path of treatment. We consider what is helpful and what does not work. We follow John as he struggles to walk his difficult and precarious path up the mountain, where each twist and turn is guaranteed to present new challenges. Some of these challenges will obviously be physical. John also has to confront feelings of isolation and despair. For her part, Beth has to come to grips with the psychological exhaustion that accompanies caretaking, an exhaustion that is rarely recognized.

We will also see how John decides to make use of alternative therapies to promote his well-being and help him cope with the physical and emotional challenges he faces in cancer treatment.

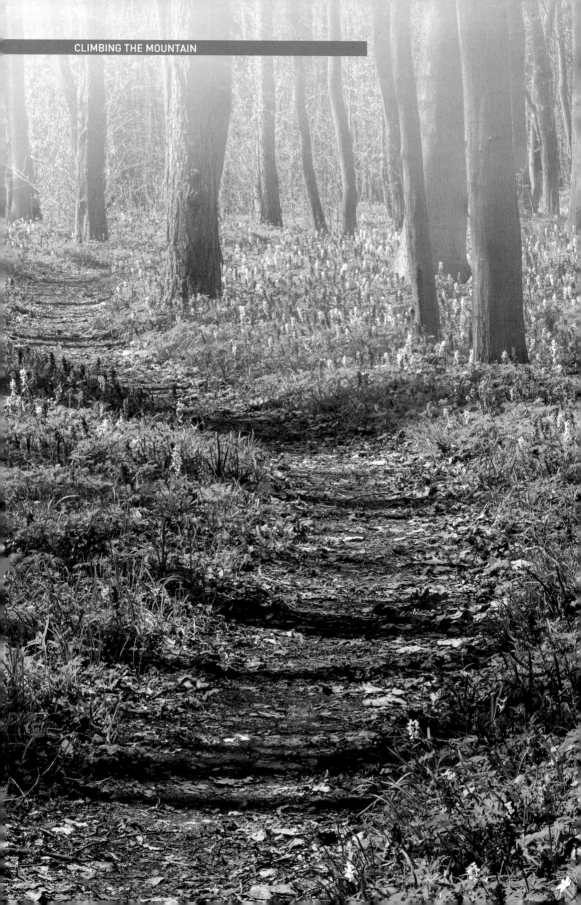

PART TWO:

Treatment

PART TWO:

Treatment

In this part of the book, we discuss the factors that influence the experience of active cancer treatment. In most cases, treatment consists of a combination of chemotherapy, immunotherapy, or radiation. The first three chapters focus on what happens in the treatment room. In Chapter 6, we look at the centrality of rituals during treatment. How and why do people perform secular rites (like wearing a lucky sweater) or religious practice (like prayer) when they visit a treatment site? In Chapter 7, we describe the sense of camaraderie that develops during treatment sessions. This social connectedness makes the treatment experience a bit easier to bear. In Chapter 8, we focus on the importance of the relations that develop between oncology nurses, who administer most cancer treatment, and patients. In Chapters 9, 10, 11, and 12, we discuss alternative activities (meditation, yoga, massage and reflexology, and social support) that can lift some of the physical and emotional difficulties that are brought on through cancer treatment. In Chapter 13, we describe how the end of treatment often triggers episodes of depression. In all of the chapters, we continue to follow John on his trek up the mountain and list some resources for readers who are interested in rituals, meditation, yoga, massage, and support groups.

6 TREATMENT RITUALS

What could be more frightening than the start of cancer treatment? Treatment usually consists of various combinations of surgery (cutting it out), radiation (burning it away), or chemotherapy (poisoning it). There are also a variety of immunotherapies that trigger the immune system to kill cancer cells. These, of course, have scary side effects. By necessity, cancer patients must subject themselves to a long and painful regimen of treatment. It is treatment that may or may not lead to a cure; perhaps it will only lead to remission or to a slow, painful descent toward death.

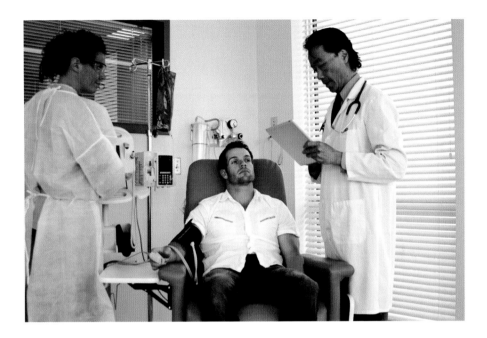

Facing the mountain of cancer treatment, with its cliffs of pain and crevasses of uncertainty, can make a cancer patient's world spin faster and faster. Patients often feel that they have lost control of their lives. How can we retain a measure of control over such a situation? What is helpful? In this chapter, we will discuss measures that provide some degree of comfort and control. They are by no means the only options available; each person, of course, has his or her own way of managing the struggle with cancer.

THE IMPORTANCE OF RITUAL

Human beings have long used rituals to give themselves a sense of control in uncontrollable circumstances. Subsistence farmers make sacrifices to the land to ensure its fertility. They make offerings to the spirits that control clouds and the wind to enhance the possibility that rain will fall on their fields. When a child becomes seriously ill, family members may engage in the ritual of prayer. Faced with a difficult challenge, human beings carry ritual objects—a rabbit's foot, a four-leaf clover, a special ring or bracelet, a particular passage found in a Chinese fortune cookie, a lucky pair of shoes or socks. Although these ritual objects may not offer physical protection from adverse elements, they provide a sense of comfort in uncomfortable situations. The anthropologist Paul Connerton (1989, 59) defined ritual as a performance that is formal "...in the sense that its structure and content are conservative and repetitive." Connerton also said that many rituals are verbal, but some "...are encoded in set postures, gestures and movement."

Cancer patients who are undergoing treatment often perform a wide variety of rituals prior to, during, and after treatment sessions. Some have a special route to follow on their way to the treatment center. Others want to sit in a particular easy chair to receive their chemotherapy drugs, or bring a lucky piece of cloth to put on their laps or to spread out on a small table next to their easy chairs. Because treatment sessions tend to last many hours, patients might find it soothing to bring particular books or special music that provide a degree of comfort during long and difficult hours. They might choose to wear special ritual objects or carry them in their pockets. Most people engage in some form of comforting ritual. Cancer treatment is a time to make use of any activity that might help ease stress and anxiety.

THE FEAR OF FIRST TREATMENT

Before his first treatment, John felt terrified. Given the range of possible side effects he had read about, he didn't know if he was more worried about his illness or what the treatment might do to him. Would he lose his hair, develop mouth sores, and experience extreme fatigue? Would he slip into depression and lose what remained of his enthusiasm and zest for life? One thing was certain: John realized that he had lost his grip on the future—at least the near future.

"What can we do, John, to make this easier for you?" Beth asked him several times.

"I don't know," he answered. "I'm worried, and I don't want to be transformed into a frail and frightened person who cannot enjoy his day-to-day life. But is that the only option?"

John and Beth decided the best course of action was to live as "normally" as possible and to enjoy as much of each day as possible under these new circumstances they faced.

"Let's take the scenic route to the treatment center—the road that follows the river. I love that drive," Beth suggested as she prepared to drive John to his first treatment.

"I am going to wear my lucky shirt." John added. "You know, the old one that I like to wear golfing, and some comfortable baggy pants."

John also had a pair of "lucky" socks. He brought his iPad so that he could listen to his favorite music—jazz and blues. When he was in high school, John played in a rock and roll band, but when he went to college, the band disbanded. Instead of playing music in college, John went to jazz and blues clubs to listen to tunes. Music had always been a big part of his life. He met Beth, in fact, at a jazz club.

John and Beth drove in silence to the treatment center. When they arrived, John signed in, and a nurse took a sample of his blood to check the levels of white and red blood cells. Eventually she led him back to an examination room to consult with Fred, his oncologist. In a calm and competent manner, Fred explained what was going to happen, describing the process and once again reviewing the possible side effects. Both John and Beth appreciated Fred's thoroughness. The treatment session would last five hours.

"Five hours?" Beth exclaimed. "What takes so long?"

"The kind of drug we're giving to John takes a long time to administer. We need to make sure that he doesn't have a severe allergic reaction."

John spent the next five hours sitting in a comfortable chair in a room filled with other cancer patients who were also receiving chemotherapy. He managed to endure his first five-hour chemotherapy-immunotherapy session. He coped by listening to his favorite music, sleeping a bit, and occasionally chatting with other patients. At some point, the nurse administered a dose of Benadryl to guard against an allergic reaction to the immunotherapy drug .The Benadryl made him drowsy. He drifted off into a dreamlike space in which he thought about old friends and the places he and his family visited—the Grand Canyon, Mount Rushmore, Atlantic City, and Europe.

The first treatment session surprised John. Like most people, he had expected a painful, difficult ordeal. Instead, he found it somewhat relaxing in a strange way. Like most people, John's life had been busy. As a lawyer, he had had a full, hectic schedule. But now the process of chemotherapy forced him to slow down not only for treatment, but also for his health and future well-being. As his treatment proceeded, John gradually developed a series of small rituals that helped him along the way.

He always took the scenic route to the treatment center. He always listened to his favorite music. Concentrating on a Chico Hamilton tune, he discovered new, nuanced elements of the music. When he listened to Eddie Harris, he let the music carry him away to a new place. He spent time remembering his past experiences. He thought about old friends and adventures. As the nurses unhooked him from his IVs, they would wish him a good evening, he would do his best to have one.

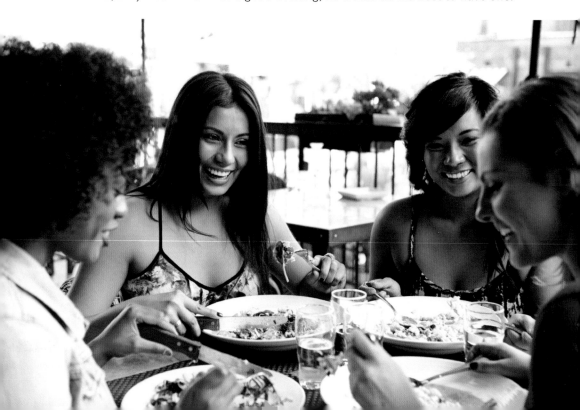

After sitting in his treatment chair for such a long time, his body would feel weak and stiff. The drugs made his limbs feel heavy. He would walk slowly to his car.

When they arrived home after John's first treatment, Beth suggested to they walk to a corner restaurant and eat a light meal. The idea of doing something as normal as eating out appealed to John.

"Let's see how you feel," Beth said. "If you are up for it, it might bring a bit of normality to a strange and difficult day. Let's try not to let cancer rule our lives. You may be getting treatment every three weeks, but after each session, if possible, we'll make it our ritual to go out to eat. That way, we take a small measure of control of our lives. If you are not up to it, we'll stay home." Beth didn't want John to feel pressured to behave normally.

RITUALS IN CANCER TREATMENT

Like John, many cancer patients rely on a variety of rituals to help them cope with the difficulties they face. Some of these are personal and some are religious. In many cases, rituals can help to ease the psychological and physical burdens of confronting cancer. Rituals can be private or shared with another person or group. Some rituals, like the ones John engaged in, involve infusing into the treatment routine ordinary day-to-day experiences that are particularly meaningful. Other people may choose to engage in more dramatic types of rituals. The importance of any ritual is the comfort it provides the person.

John found that listening to music provided him with the greatest sense of comfort during his treatments. He found that this was not unusual. Music appeared to be a useful way for many people to cope with difficult treatments. His research indicated that music therapy helped promote healing and improved one's quality of life. John also read that music therapy helped promote emotional expression during difficult times and that it helped relieve treatment symptoms. In fact, John read that music was helpful in relieving the pain and nausea associated with chemotherapy. He was grateful that he had always appreciated music and that he could benefit from that appreciation during this painful period of his life.

John also read that music therapy had the additional benefits of lowering one's heart rate and blood pressure. Although John hoped that his treatment would be effective, he also learned that a music practice called music thanatology could be used to help a person at the end of life. The ancient Greek philosophers believed that music could heal not only the body but also the soul. In Native American and various African societies, ritual singing and dancing played major roles in the healing processes. For these reasons, John always listened to his music during his treatments. Music gave him comfort, eased his pain, and took him to a different place with sunshine and fresh air.

http://www.cancer.org/treatment/treatmentsandsideeffects/complementaryandalternativemedicine/mindbodyandspirit/music-therapy

Below is a list of some books and websites that discuss the role of ritual in the cancer experience.

1. Muschal-Reinhardt, Rosalie, Mitrano, Barbara S., McCarthy, Mary Rose, Grinnan, Jeanne Brinkman. 2000. *Rituals for Women Coping With Breast Cancer.* Orange County, CA: The Prism Collective.
2. Jeannine Walston, *Ritual and Cancer.* http://jeanninewalston.com/integrative-cancer-care/spirit/ritual-and-cancer/
3. *Mind, Body, and Spirit.* American Cancer Society www.cancer.org, Nov 1, 2008. This piece focuses on religion, spirituality, herbal medicine, and rituals that Native Americans perform for cancer as well as other diseases.
4. Buchbinder, M., Longofter, J. and McCue, K. 2009. "Family routines and rituals when a parent has cancer." *Fam Syst Health.* 2009 Sep; 27(3): 213-27.
5. *Meditation and Cancer Rituals.* http://ritualsofhealing.com/cancersupport/
6. www.researchgate.net/.../259455996_The_role_of_complementary medicine in men's cancer treatment.
7. Dein, Simon. 2005. *Culture and Cancer Care: Anthropological Insights in Oncology.* New York: McGraw Hill.

8.   Connerton, Paul. 1989. *How Societies Remember*. Cambridge: Cambridge University Press.

9.   Turner, Victor. 1969. *The Ritual Process: Structure and Anti-Structure.* Ithaca, NY: Cornell University Press.

There is no one ritual for any set of cancer treatments. There is also no one ritual that can take the cancer patient away from the unpleasantness of treatment. But there are a wide variety of rituals we can perform to ease the burden of treatment. The best strategy is to find rituals that match our personal sensibilities. For some people like John, in addition to listening to music, it might mean wearing a particular watch or article of clothing, or taking a special route to the treatment center. For other people, it might mean participating in group activities like guided meditation, or rites, like sweat lodges, fashioned from Native American ceremonial life. Many people find prayer helpful.

Whatever ritual we choose, we shouldn't feel embarrassed or foolish. Human beings have been performing rituals for tens of thousands of years, for two very good reasons. First, they connect us to others in times of need. Second, they provide a sense of control in stressful situations. In short, rituals are woven tightly into the fabric of human existence. They give us peace and hope when we are sick.

7 CAMARADERIE IN THE TREATMENT ROOM

As stated in the previous chapter, rituals provide cancer patients with a measure of comfort in an uncomfortable situation. They offer a degree of control in a situation that is, to a large extent, uncontrollable. The power of ritual enables cancer patients to walk with a slightly steadier gait on the path that leads up the mountain. But there are other comforting dimensions of ritual that patients undergoing treatment may experience. One of these is the solidarity and camaraderie that may develop in a cancer treatment room.

TREATMENT BONDING

Scholars have long written about such camaraderie. Anthropologists Victor and Edith Turner, for example, who were pioneers of the anthropology of ritual, called such a special feeling of connectedness "communitas." Here's what Edith Turner says about this phenomenon in her 2012 book, *Communitas, the Anthropology of Collective Joy.*

> ...The characteristics of communitas show it to be almost beyond strict definition, with almost endless variations. Communitas often appears unexpectedly. It has to do with a sense felt by a group of people when their life together takes on full meaning....Communitas can only be conveyed through stories....(p.1)

She goes on to say that:

> This book...tackles communitas, togetherness itself, taking the reader to the edge of the precipice of knowledge—and beyond, over the barrier of the scientists' analysis and into experience itself. Light dawns on what the real thing is, and we feel lucky it exists. Then we can make discoveries. (p. 11).

This feeling of camaraderie is also evident in the 2013 film *50/50*, in which a young man, Adam, only 28 years old, is diagnosed with a rare form of cancer and given a 50/50 chance of survival. Numbed by his sudden and completely unexpected confrontation with mortality, he is understandably frightened when he checks in for his first chemotherapy treatment. As he slips into an easy chair and a nurse connects him to an IV, Adam meets two men who greet him with surprisingly good cheer. One of the men passes him a bag full of brownies.

My wife baked them, he says. They're laced with medical marijuana. Helps me get through these long chemo sessions.

They are really good, the other man says.

Adam says that he's never smoked marijuana and would prefer to pass. The men are insistent and Adam eats a brownie. He gets high as he sails through his first chemotherapy session. At the same time, Adam forges a bond with these other men who are, in many ways, sharing his experience—the fear, the uncertainty, and the disorientation, as well as the emotional and physical pain. Adam's situation is not unique.

THE IMPORTANCE OF PATIENT LEARNING

Like most cancer patients, John began his treatment with considerable fear and trepidation. He was worried about many things, including the physical impact of the side effects of toxic chemotherapy drugs. Would he be continuously nauseous? Would he lose his taste for food? Would he lose weight? Would he lose all of his hair? Would he develop painful mouth sores? And what about fatigue? Would he have the energy to drive his car, work, and spend time with his family and friends? And what about bone pain and numbness in his fingers and feet—all possible side effects of chemotherapy drugs? How would he cope if he experienced some or all of these?

John read everything he could on the physical and emotional impact of chemotherapy. He learned what kind of questions to ask his physician. He knew enough to make informed choices about his treatment. Even so, the prospect of a prolonged period of fatigue, pain, and physical transformation made him fear for his life—even more than his initial diagnosis did.

After his first chemotherapy session, though, he felt better. He realized that he was not alone in this new challenge he was facing. From the outset of his treatment he felt a bond with the other patients in the treatment room. While hooked up to his IV, he looked around the treatment room and realized that his fellow patients came from every segment of society. Some were older; others were younger. A worried-looking father from South Asia sat by his teenaged daughter as chemotherapy agents dripped into her body. An equal number of men and women received treatment that day. Some sat by themselves, reading a book or listening to music; others talked quietly with family members or friends. Some of the patients looked like they were prosperous; others appeared to be poor. One older man, who said he had been an electrician, worried about his co-payment increasing,

"If it goes up anymore," he told the nurse, "I won't be able to continue my treatments."

"Don't worry, Harry," another patient said. "There are programs. We can always help you."

Like the patient in the film 50/50, John would have been grateful for some medical marijuana to help him through his first chemotherapy session. Marijuana (THC) has been proven to have anti-inflammatory benefits. It is also known to help with chronic pain and appears to be safer than opioids. More information on the benefits of medical marijuana can be found at the following website:

(http://medicalmarijuana.procon.org/view.resource.php?resourceID=000881). Indeed, the legal use of medical marijuana is on the rise.

Although John did not have medical marijuana available to him, he quickly began to feel at ease with his fellow patients. Somehow, the knowledge that his fellow patients were all trekking up the mountain—all facing similar sets of issues—made chemotherapy a bit easier to bear.

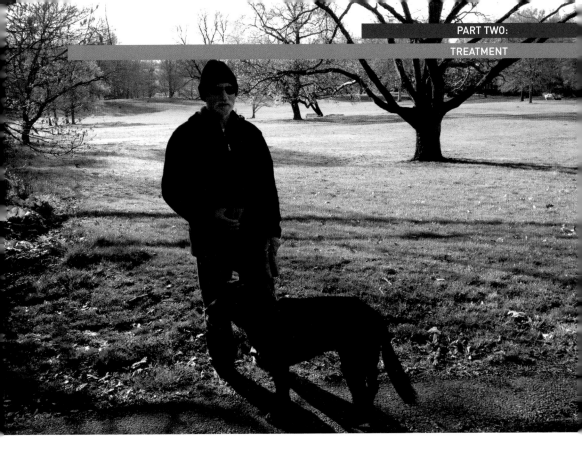

JOHN'S DAY IN TREATMENT

The nurses at the Cancer Center usually scheduled John's treatments for 10:00 a.m. On treatment days he would wake up at 7:00 in the morning, have a cup of tea with Beth, and eat a light breakfast. Then he would take a two-mile walk with his dog. He knew that after treatment he would not have enough energy for such activity.

During the walk John would try to focus on his physical surroundings instead of what he was facing later in the day. When he got home, he would get ready, and Beth would drive him to the Cancer Center. John needed to arrive 15 minutes before the start of treatment for blood work to make certain that his blood cell counts were good enough to proceed to treatment. If the counts proved to be good, a nurse would call his name and would accompany him to the treatment room, a rectangular space with lots of windows through which abundant sunlight streaked.

In that space, the staff arranged a collection of easy chairs in alcoves formed with mobile partitions, which meant that no one received chemotherapy in physical isolation. Then the nurse would insert a needle into a vein (sometimes a challenge) in his wrist and hook him up to a chemo drip. After approximately one hour of the drip, the nurse would give him a 25-mg infusion of Benadryl. Following the Benadryl, John would have to sit through a four-hour slow drip of an immunotherapy drug, which was necessary because of the possibility of a severe allergic reaction.

At the outset of treatment John might read, but once the Benadryl took effect, he let his music carry him into hazy sleep and hopefully a good dream. During his good dreams, he found himself travelling back to his past. He thought of old friends and of places where he adventured as a young man. He re-lived his honeymoon. He imagined himself as healthy and adventurous, peacefully rowing in a canoe on a river or a tributary. The Benadryl took him to comforting places, and then, as the effects gradually wore off, it gently provided him a soft landing in his easy chair.

BONDING PROCESSES

The anthropologist Victor Turner's description of people in between things aptly describes the feeling of being in limbo that John and other cancer patients often experience. Like anyone who finds himself or herself in the between,

> They tend to be humble and follow instructions without complaint—the cancer patient following the advice for combating the side effects of chemotherapy drugs. They tend to accept regimes of pain—the cancer patient authorizing a course of chemotherapy, surgery, or radiation. They are reduced to a common denominator, the 'cancer patient,' so they might be reconstructed. These processes…trigger an intense camaraderie, which undermines previously recognized differences in age, social status, and ethnicity. (Stoller 2008, 146)

During his treatments John would have conversations with whoever happened to be sitting close to him. Given that he was often on a similar schedule as others, he gradually got to know his fellow patients. There was Suzanne, the forty-something teacher who was receiving treatment for breast cancer. He liked talking to her husband and sister when they visited during her treatment time. Her prognosis was good, and she was feeling optimistic about her illness. There was another patient named John who was not optimistic about his future but attempted to keep up a good front. There were younger and older men and women of different backgrounds. John was grateful for their conversation, for the camaraderie, for the shared feeling, for being able to talk openly about his illness. He had already learned that although he had supportive friends, it was difficult for them to know what to say when he discussed his illness.

The bond with his fellow patients was one of the factors that made John's treatment bearable. For him, the treatment room became a community of people sharing a difficult life experience.

SUGGESTIONS FOR FURTHER READING AND VIEWING

1. Summit Entertainment, Mandate Pictures and Point Grey Pictures. 2012. *50/50*. 100 minutes.
2. Stoller, Paul. 2008. *The Power of the Between*. Chicago: The University of Chicago Press.
3. Stoller, Paul. 2013. "Cancer Rites and the Remission Society." *Harvard Divinity Bulletin* 41: 69-71.
4. Turner, Victor. 1969. *The Ritual Process: Structure and Anti-Structure*. New York: Cornell University Press.

8 NURSE-PATIENT RELATIONSHIPS

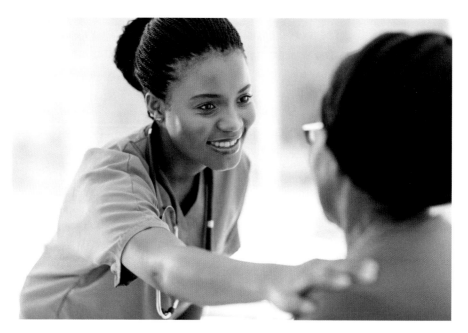

From the time of diagnosis to the beginning of treatment, cancer patients interact with a variety of medical professionals: medical oncologists, radiologists, oncological surgeons, and technicians who do ultrasounds, CT scans, PET scans, and blood work. Such an array of cancer professionals sometimes obscures the primary importance of the oncology nurse—the principal player in cancer treatment.

Oncology nurses escort nervous patients from waiting areas to treatment rooms. They make sure that patients are comfortable in their easy chairs. They mix chemotherapy medicines, making sure that the medicines and doses are correct. If they make an error, it would have serious, if not fatal consequences. Given the circumstances of their work with patients who are dealing, for the most part, with illnesses that have no cure, they tend to be remarkably pleasant and empathetic. They know their patients on a very personal level. They know their patients in ways that other medical personnel cannot.

Oncology nurses are the professionals who hook us up to the IV line that will carry chemotherapy or immunotherapy drugs into the blood stream. Many of the nurses are quite skilled at inserting a needle into a hand or wrist vein. They are delicate about inserting a line into a chest port for those patients who receive more regular chemotherapy treatments. If an oncology nurse says that he or she is going to look after you, then you are very lucky indeed. Good oncology nurses can transform a very stressful and fearful situation into a bearable one.

Being a nurse is one of the most demanding occupations imaginable, and being an oncology nurse increases that stress. In fact, nursing has been found to be an occupation that leads to a high rate of overload and burnout. Dealing with physicians and patients (often patients who are coping with unimaginable difficulties) makes life difficult. Research has indicated that feeling overloaded and coping with patient suffering leads to considerable stress among nurses. In one study of 35 oncology nurses, 50 percent stated that work situations were stressful, and 22 percent felt extremely stressed (http://www.ncbi.nlm.nih.gov/pubmed/15915061).

Oncology nurses are highly trained professionals who are continuously developing their skills to keep up with new developments in cancer treatment.

Many oncology nurses conduct research, hold administration positions, teach at nursing schools, and provide direct patient care. These specialists are employed in all medical settings, including hospitals, consulting firms, cancer treatment facilities, doctors' offices, assisted living facilities, veterans' hospitals, and any other facility where cancer patients receive treatment. Oncology nurses also manage care, discuss patients' conditions with physicians and other cancer specialists, and coordinate treatments for recovering patients.

Advanced practitioners supervise patient care, evaluate staff member performance, meet with family members of cancer victims, and occasionally provide diagnoses.

Oncology nurses working as coordinators are responsible for organizing and managing treatment. Often, they're responsible for overseeing the efforts of multiple specialists working in teams. When managing care, coordinators must set attainable goals for patients.

Oncology nurses are required to be registered nurses with specialized training. They must complete training to become acquainted with basic cancer treatment knowledge and skills. Additionally, they must obtain some clinical experience beyond what is acquired in general nursing training programs.

[http://www.collegeatlas.org/oncology-nurse.html]

JOHN'S NURSES

Before being diagnosed with cancer, John had not given much thought to the social world of medicine—the divides among physicians, medical administrators, nurses, medical technicians, and medical staff. As John encountered these various professionals, he developed a great deal of respect for them. But among the dedicated practitioners John encountered, he came to respect the work of the oncology nurses the most. As they monitored his chemotherapy treatments, these men and women tended to maintain a cheerful countenance. They patiently and attentively listened to the expression of patient fears and concerns. They monitored active treatment intervention, intervening if problems developed. They tended to patients who needed comfort. In short, the oncology nurses provided John and his fellow patients both professional treatment and a considerable degree of comfort and solace.

Over time John established friendly relationships with several of his nurses. They were nice to him. He talked to them about his family and work. They asked after his dog. They became an important factor that helped to make his once-every-three-weeks, five-hour treatment sessions easier to bear. The nurses also took the time to talk to John about how to manage life between treatments. They had considerable knowledge about how treatment shaped the quality of life. They talked with John about his activities and asked him about his stress level. They wondered how he had attempted to cope with the stress he felt. They encouraged him to stay as active as possible. The nurses were doing more than just treating John's disease and treatment side effects. They treated John like a person. John continuously expressed his gratitude for their help and suggestions.

"No matter how fatigued you are, John," one nurse told him, "Try to go the gym, even just for a few moments. If that doesn't work, take a walk and get some fresh air. Activity will make you feel better and give you a sense of normality."

As much as possible, John followed this excellent advice. Although the chemotherapy made him heavy with fatigue, he was always able to take a short walk outside or occasionally go to the gym.

Beyond all the well-meaning advice he received from his family and friends and the knowledge he had gleaned from his research and reading, it was often the advice of his nurses that was the most on target. It was often their advice that motivated him to try a new activity that might enhance the quality of his life. The nurses who helped to administer his treatments had gained considerable knowledge about what helped patients manage their illness. What's more, they also helped to make the long hours in the treatment room a bit more bearable.

In some ways, John was lucky. In recent decades, both physicians and nurses have consciously worked to improve their communication with patients. Medical training has increasingly focused on communication skills and on understanding the whole person rather than simply his or her illness. Studies have found that satisfying communication between nurses and their patients can make a significant difference in how well a patient copes with his or her illness. Clearly teaching future doctors and nurses how to create a clinical climate of empathy is an important element of medical training. One of the cornerstones of the patient–nurse relationship revolves around the nurse's ability to be empathetic with the patient. Empathy is defined as being aware of, sensitive to, and vicariously experiencing the feelings of another.

John's nurses listened to their patients. They joked and laughed in difficult and painful situations. They dealt forthrightly with treatment successes and failures. No matter the circumstance, they maintained their humanity.

ADDITIONAL RESOURCES ON ONCOLOGY NURSE–PATIENT RELATIONS

1. Price, Diana 2014. *Uncommon Bonds: Oncology Nurses and Patients.* http://awomanshealth.com/uncommon-bonds-oncology-nurses-and-patients/
2. Vahid Zamanzadeh, Roghaieh Azimzadeh, Azad Rahmani and Leila Valizadeh. *Oncology patients' and professional nurses' perceptions of important nurse caring behaviors.* http://www.biomedcentral.com/1472-6955/9/10.
3. Bauer, Bauer. 2014. *Spotlight On: Oncology Nurses – Part I, a Q&A.* http://www.cancer.net/blog/2014-05/spotlight-oncology-nurses-%E2%80%93-part-i-qa.
4. Coffey, Sue. 2006. The Nurse–Patient Relationship in Cancer Care as a Shared Covenant. *Advances in Nursing Science* Vol. 29, No. 4, pp. 308–323

9 MEDITATION

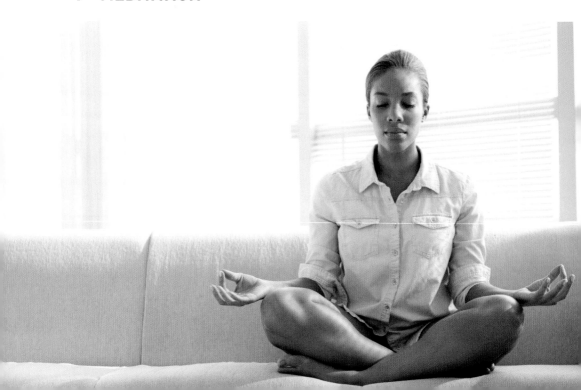

As treatment proceeds, the side effects of chemotherapy tend to increase. John was no exception. As his treatment progressed, he managed to adjust to the discomforts and weakness associated with chemotherapy. In many respects, he was lucky. He didn't lose his hair. Although he didn't have debilitating nausea, he did feel achy and weak. Despite the privations of treatment, John was able to engage in a reduced version of his everyday life. Even so, he still hoped to find ways that would enable him to live more fully during his treatment. He and Beth researched the various options available and found a considerable amount of research in support of meditation.

THE PATH OF MEDITATION

According to the information that John and Beth discovered, regular meditation practice reduced stress and increased "mindfulness." It lowered blood pressure and helped boost the immune system to fight infection and disease. Recent research on mindfulness demonstrated that regular meditation not only reduced stress and increased physical well-being but also seemed to have a physical impact at the cellular level.

Meditation has been practiced for thousands of years. The earliest records of mediation are from India. Herbert Benson conducted one of the early studies that explored the physiological changes that occur during meditation. He found that it eased high blood pressure. Numerous studies have since supported the health-promoting effects of regular meditation.

In a *Huffington Post* blog post published on November 5, 2014, Carolyn Gregoire wrote:

Mindfulness meditation is known to have a positive emotional and psychological impact on cancer survivors. But some groundbreaking new research has found that meditation is also doing its work on the physical bodies of cancer survivors, with positive impacts extending down to the cellular level.

Practicing mindfulness meditation or being involved in a social support group causes positive cellular changes in breast cancer survivors, according to researchers at Alberta Health Services and the University of Calgary. (http://www.huffingtonpost.com/2014/11/05/mindfulness-meditation-cancer_n_6101130.html)

According to Project Meditation, there are widespread physical and psychological benefits that emerge from regular meditation.

According to reports, there have been over 1500 separate studies since 1930. All were related to meditation and its effects on the practitioners. Some statistics on people who meditate show that:

+ Heart rate, respiration, blood pressure, and oxygen consumption were all decreased.
+ Meditators were less anxious and nervous.
+ Meditators were more independent and self-confident.
+ People who meditated daily were less fearful of death.
+ 75 percent of insomniacs who started a daily meditation program were able to fall asleep within 20 minutes of going to bed.
+ Production of the stress hormone cortisol was greatly decreased, thus making it possible for those people to deal with stress better when it occurred.
+ Women with PMS showed symptom improvements after 5 months of steady daily rumination and reflection.
+ Thickness of the artery walls decreased, which effectively lowers the risk of heart attack or stroke by 8 to 15 percent.
+ Relaxation therapy was helpful in chronic pain patients.
+ 60 percent of anxiety-prone people showed marked improvements in anxiety levels after 6 to 9 months.

Meditation may even serve as a "Fountain of Youth." It has been documented that people who regularly use meditation and relaxation techniques may be physiologically younger by 12 to 15 years. Could this possibly be true? The research results are vast and multifaceted. In general, the results suggest that meditation (or relaxation, reflection, and deliberation) can affect the physical body in positive ways, just as stress and other factors affect the body in negative ways. In either case, it is clear that scientific studies of people who regularly mediate confirm the positive effects of meditation (http://www.project-meditation.org/a_wim1/statistics_on_people_who_meditate.html).

In one important study conducted in 2012, researchers found that "African Americans with heart disease who practiced Transcendental Meditation regularly were 48 percent less likely to have a heart-attack, stroke or die from all causes compared with African Americans who attended a health education class for more than five years, according to new research published in the American Heart Association journal Circulation: *Cardiovascular Quality and Outcomes*." (http://www.sciencedaily.com/releases/2012/11/121113161504.htm)

Cancer centers are even beginning to offer meditation as "alternative" medicine. In a 2011 blog post, Dr. Joseph Nowinski wrote about the usefulness of meditation as a support for cancer treatment:

> There is good news when it comes to meditation as a complementary treatment, and that is that a number of rigorous clinical trials are underway. Using controlled clinical trials, these investigators are studying the effects of both types of meditation on health issues such as hypertension, cardiovascular disease and the side effects of cancer treatment. The common denominator driving this research is a general recognition that chronic stress is linked to a variety of health problems, such as increased heart disease, compromised immune system functioning and premature cellular and cognitive aging. It makes sense, then, to take a closer look at how meditation can help. Here is a sample of what researchers have discovered and verified so far:

+ A study of 60 breast cancer survivors found that women who practiced meditation reduced the number and severity of hot flashes and also reported improvements in mood and sleep.
+ A study of 63 people with rheumatoid arthritis found that mindfulness

> meditation helped to improve quality of life and reduce psychological
> distress.
>
> + A study of 298 college students found that transcendental meditation
>   helped students reduce stress and improve coping strategies.
> + A "meta-analysis" of 10 studies found that mindfulness meditation
>   improves the overall mental health of cancer patients. (Huffington
>   Post, May 10, 2011)

There are many articles in prestigious medical journals that incontrovertibly reference the positive psychological benefits of regular meditation to anyone, including, of course cancer patients. Why is it, then, that only a small percentage of the American adult population practices meditation? In a 2013 study, Williams et al. wrote: "National surveys indicate only a small segment of the United States population practices meditation (Barnes, Bloom, & Nahin, 2008). The most recent National Health Interview Survey (n = 23,393) found prevalence of use for meditation in the general adult population is approximately 9%" (Nursing Research 61(1): 22).

In one study on this topic, the authors discussed the most important barriers to regular meditative practice: the absence of a quiet space and general feelings of restlessness (such as not being able to sit still for 10, 15, or 20 minutes). The authors bypass the broader cultural barriers to a more widespread practice of meditation. The general pace of life in North America and Europe is fast-paced. People complain about not having time enough to relax, and when they are on vacation, they are often worried about what they are missing at work. Work conditions are also making Americans more and more stressed. A 2013 *Huffington Post* article reported on the results of a new survey:

A new survey shows that more than 8 in 10 employed Americans are stressed out by at least one thing about their jobs. Poor pay and increasing workloads were top sources of concern reported by American workers. The third annual Work Stress Survey, conducted by Harris Interactive on behalf of Everest College, polled 1,019 employed Americans by phone. The results showed a marked increase from last year's survey, which found that 73 percent of Americans were stressed at work.

This year that number jumped to 83 percent. Only 17 percent of workers said that nothing about their jobs causes them stress (http://www.huffingtonpost.com/2013/04/10/work-stress-jobs-americans_n_3053428.html).

Workers, or at least American workers, are expected to do more and more in an atmosphere of intense competition and the ever-present threat of job loss. This atmosphere has come about in an era of market fundamentalism in which the economic forces of the market celebrate the warrior who assesses, competes, wins, and dominates. In such a space there is little time to engage in philosophical conversation or directed inner reflection. There is less time to secure a calm space to engage in regular meditation.

Another barrier to the promotion of meditation among cancer patients lies in the predominant philosophy of the medical establishment when it comes to the treatment of cancer. The warrior identity is central to the cancer experience as well. Although oncologists are making more space for complementary medicine, the governing metaphor in the medical world—including the world of cancer—is immunology, in which the establishment (physicians, nurses, and patients) must wage war (surgery, radiation, drugs) to conquer disease and then dominate it. As a cancer patient, it is not uncommon to hear people say:

"You can beat this."

"You need to be a fighter."

"Be strong. Don't give up."

In contemporary times, we are rewarded for drive, ambition, and competitive edge. In social terms, we are not rewarded for our inner sensitivity, the capacity to converse, or the tranquility of our inner being, all of which helps to explain why such a small percentage of people practice the health-promoting techniques of meditation.

To reiterate, meditation is the most widely used mind-body therapy among Americans. In one study, almost 10 percent of Americans, or 20 million people, had practiced some form of meditation. Meditation consists of a variety of practices focusing on relaxation and stress relief. Meditation is an ancient contemplative practice that has received considerable interest in social science research. According to the aforementioned studies, it provides relief from anxiety, helps ease depression, increases attention and memory, and helps improve sleep patterns (http://www.huffingtonpost.com/2014/10/15/scientific-american-meditation_n_5991084.html).

JOHN TRIES MEDITATION

After conducting research on the benefits of meditation, John felt that he could not go wrong. It was certainly worth a try. Before his cancer diagnosis, John, like the majority of Americans, knew little about meditation. Being a "baby boomer," John had heard about meditation, but he associated meditation with the 1960 "hippie" era during which thousands of young Americans went to India to be enlightened. The most common path to enlightenment was Transcendental Meditation (TM).

Prior to his cancer diagnosis, John, as we have seen, had a busy and active life. He had always tried to maintain a sense of balance and felt that he had usually been successful. When he was diagnosed with cancer, however, the balance shifted. His life had been turned upside down. As his treatment proceeded, this feeling increased. After several chemotherapy sessions, John's oncology nurse suggested that he try meditation. She knew that he had been researching the benefits of complementary treatment methods. Several patients, she told him, had greatly benefited from meditation. She felt certain it would help John.

John had a great deal of respect for this kind nurse. Her encouragement combined with his research findings made him decide to try meditation. The nurse found a card that listed the address of a conveniently located yoga/meditation center in town and gave it to John. "The people are very nice," she told John, "and I have seen the space. It's very peaceful and beautiful."

John took the information and began his journey on the path of meditation. Before he signed up for a class, he conducted further research on his options. He and Beth found out that the Center offered two kinds of meditation: concentrative (CM) and mindful (MM).

In CM, you learn how to focus on a single sound, mantra, or perhaps an image and let that concentration carry you away on a meditative journey. In MM, you learn to become conscious of all of your thoughts and perceptions, letting them move in and out of your mind. In this way, you learn to empty your mind and let go.

"Let's try CM," Beth, who had decided to join John, suggested. "We can go to class together and see if we like it. If CM doesn't work out, we'll try the other technique."

Several days after John signed them up for a meditation session, they walked up the steps to the top floor of a pleasant-looking two-story building. John pushed open the double doors at the top of the stairs and they entered a dimly lit rectangular room with a hardwood floor. Mats and meditation pillows had been positioned in one corner of the windowless room. The facilitator, a tall, thin woman with long gray hair, welcomed them. Soothing Indian music pulsed softly in the background.

"Take a mat and a pillow, and get comfortable."

Other meditators slowly made their way up the stairs. They gathered their mats and pillows and quietly greeted John and Beth. The facilitator rang a bell and began to talk softly to the group of about 20 people. "Welcome, friends. We'll stretch a bit and get ourselves loose and then we'll begin to meditate." They stretched their arms, backs, and legs for about 15 minutes, and then the facilitator asked everyone to sit on their pillows.

"We'll do some exercises called alternate nostril breathing. You breathe in through your right nostril and use your finger to compress the left nostril and vice versa."

John proceeded with this exercise and began to feel relaxed, and a physical sense of well-being came over him—something that had eluded him during his cancer treatment.

The facilitator continued. "Okay, now I want you to close your eyes. Inhale deeply, and silently say the number '1' when you exhale. Then inhale, and when you exhale, say '2,' and so on until you reach 20. When you reach '20,' do the same thing, counting back down to 1. Begin when I ring the bell. Take your time and just let the process unfold."

John had been doubtful that the exercise would bear positive results. He went through the motions, inhaling and exhaling and slowly counting up to 20 and down to 1. By the time he got to 9, he found himself focusing on people and places from his past. He found himself in the redwood forests in California, lying on the beach, and biking through the woods. When the facilitator rang the bell to signal the end of this exercise, John felt as if he had been in a trance. He hadn't realized that 20 minutes had passed.

He turned to Beth. "That wasn't so bad."

Beth smiled and nodded. She had enjoyed the time as well. Since John had gotten sick, Beth had been anxious and worried. She was beginning to feel exhausted from John's long odyssey of treatment. Maybe meditation was something that would help her.

The facilitator continued. "As you get more and more relaxed, you might wander away. Don't fight it. If you wander on a meditative journey, we wish you a nice trip." She smiled. "Let's try one more exercise. This time, do one of two things: repeat a short phrase, or a mantra, over and over again, or concentrate on a single sound or image to the exclusion of all other images and see what happens. We'll do this exercise for 20 minutes. Before we begin, you might want to stand up and stretch your legs. When you're ready, take a seat on the pillow and make sure you're comfortable. When I ring the bell, pick your object of concentration and begin your practice."

She rang the bell.

John concentrated on the image of a peaceful beach. He closed his eyes and returned to his blanket on the beach, slowly breathing in and out. His pulse slowed down. He became conscious of his beating heart. He was so relaxed that the cross-legged, seated pose caused him no discomfort. The ringing bell brought him back to the room, back to the other meditators and back to the present with all of its anxieties. He felt calmer. He slowly got up and helped Beth to her feet. They smiled at one another.

"We should do this all the time," John suggested.

THE APPROPRIATENESS OF MEDITATION

Not everyone will have the same positive reaction as John and Beth. For some people, sitting silently for 20 or 30 minutes is difficult and uncomfortable. John and Beth were both quite pleased with the process. They decided to begin practicing at home as a supplement to the weekly class. Every morning, they meditated for 15 minutes. The benefits were immediate. Their days passed by at a more relaxed pace. They both felt that they were calmer and able to think more clearly. Beth especially felt that meditation provided her with much-needed relief. On those days when one or both of them were not able to practice, they felt that something was missing. John and Beth began to think about meditation the way some people think about prayer or exercise: if you miss one day, something is not quite right.

There is no one way to practice meditation. Meditation is designed to change how the mind works.

+ Ideally, meditation should be practiced in the morning and the evening for up to 45 minutes, but even a short 5- to 10-minute meditation session each day is helpful.
+ During meditation the mind is directed in a way to center one's attention on an object, person, emotional state, word, or phrase.
+ Mindfulness meditation is one popular form of meditation that focuses on directing attention to the present moment, the body, sounds, words, or phrases.
+ Meditation is not for everyone. Some people simply are not able to let go or relax enough to enjoy the meditative journey. But as

John's example illustrates, meditation can be very helpful during the stressful times of cancer treatment. Here are a few recent suggested readings about practices and the benefits of meditation for anyone, especially cancer patients.

1. American Cancer Society. *Meditation.* http://www. cancer.org/treatment/treatmentsandsideeffects/ complementaryandalternativemedicine/mindbodyandspirit/ meditation.

2. Eldridge, Lynn, MD. 2013. *Meditation for People With Cancer: How Can Meditation Help People Living With Cancer?* http://lungcancer. about.com/od/alternativetreatment1/a/Meditation-Cancer.htm

3. Nowinski, Joseph 2011. How Meditation Can Support Cancer Treatment. *The Huffington Post,* November 5, 2011.

4. Gregoire, Carolyn 2014. How Meditation Can Help Protect The Body After Cancer. *The Huffington Post,* November 5, 2014. http:// www.huffingtonpost.com/2014/11/05/mindfulness-meditation-cancer_n_6101130.html

5. Wong, Kathy. 2013. *Can Meditation Help With Cancer?* http:// altmedicine.about.com/od/cance1/a/meditation_cancer.htm

6. Carson, Linda, et al. 2014. Mindfulness-based cancer recovery and supportive-expressive therapy maintain telomere length relative to controls in distressed breast cancer survivors. *Oncology and Radiotherapy.* November 3. http://onlinelibrary.wiley.com/ doi/10.1002/cncr.29063/full

7. Ott, May Jane, et al. 2006. Mindfulness Meditation for Oncology Patients: A Discussion and Critical Review of Integrative *Cancer Therapies* Vol. 5 (2) 98-108.

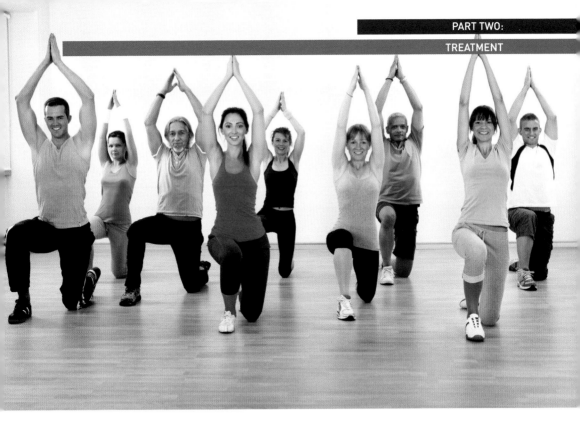

10 YOGA

During his treatment, John managed to keep going. He continued to work at his law firm, though he cut back on his hours. He and Beth took regular walks and short bike rides. Periodically they would meet friends for dinner or go to a concert. Sometimes, however, John felt weary. When he met with other cancer patients, he felt he could fully express his frustration about his lack of energy. Throughout his treatment, his daily routine of meditation helped to keep him calm.

Given the effectiveness of meditation, John decided it might be a good idea to explore additional complementary techniques. As treatment dragged on, he felt weaker from chemotherapy's side effects. Maybe it would be good to look for additional ways to stay active—something that did not completely deplete his limited energy. Several of his friends practiced yoga regularly and loved it. They encouraged John to look into this ancient practice.

THE HISTORY OF YOGA

Yoga is as old as ancient Indian civilization. Early mention of yoga can be found ancient texts like the *Upanishads* and the *Bhagavad-Gita* as well in the sacred texts of Buddhism. The classical period of yoga began in the 2nd Century ACE when Patanjali wrote the Yoga Sutra. That text consists of aphorisms about the relation among mind, body, and well-being. According to a blog written by Shanebance (an Internet ID) on the ABC's of Yoga website, classical yoga is defined through Patanjali's Eightfold Path of Yoga (also called Eight Limbs of Classical Yoga).

1. *Yama,* which means social restraints or ethical values;
2. *Niyama,* which is personal observance of purity, tolerance, and study;
3. *Asanas* or physical exercises;
4. *Pranayama,* which means breath control or regulation;
5. *Pratyahara* or sense withdrawal in preparation for Meditation;
6. *Dharana,* which is about concentration;
7. *Dhyana,* which means Meditation; and
8. *Samadhi,* which means ecstasy.

Patanjali believed that each individual is a composite of matter (*prakriti*) and spirit (*purusha*). He further believed that the two must be separated in order to cleanse the spirit, in stark contrast to Vedic and Pre-Classical Yoga, which signify the union of body and spirit (http://abc-of-yoga.com/beginnersguide/yogahistory.asp).

While yoga focuses on learning postures and increasing flexibility and strength, it has a much broader purpose. Yoga has always been about the spiritual transformation of a person. In fact, in Hinduism and Buddhism, yoga means "spiritual discipline." Yoga has been practiced for thousands of years (http://iml.jou.ufl.edu/projects/fall05/levy/history.html).

According to the National Institutes of Health, yoga is linked to a considerable number of health benefits. These include increased flexibility, coordination, balance, concentration, memory, sleep, and immune system functioning. Like meditation, yoga is also beneficial for coping with stress and anxiety and for preventing depression.

YOGA IN CONTEMPORARY TIMES

The ancient practice of yoga is widely practiced today in North America and in Europe. In the U.S., we can find a variety of yoga centers in every city and in most small towns. Yoga comes in many forms: yoga flow, meditative yoga, and, for the especially vigorous, hot yoga, during which you do a variety of poses in a studio heated well above 100 degrees Fahrenheit. According to The Yoga Journal, in 2012, roughly 8.7 percent of Americans practiced yoga regularly, which translates to 20.4 million Americans, many of whom are beginners. Billions of dollars are spent each year on yoga products and yoga lessons. There are gender and age distinctions among people who practice yoga in the United States:

+ Yogis tend to be women, accounting for 82.2 percent of respondents in the survey, and young: 62.8 percent of all respondents were between 18 and 44 years old. They're also willing to spend: American yogis shell out an estimated $10.3 billion each year on their habit, between classes, equipment, clothing, and other products.
+ Yoga practitioners state that the primary reason they started yoga was to improve physical fitness. More than three-quarters, or 78.3 percent, said they were motivated to improve flexibility. Overall conditioning, stress relief, and improved general health and fitness levels were other popular motivational factors (http://www. huffingtonpost.com/2012/12/06/american-yoga_n_2251360.html).

The physical health benefits of regular yoga practice are also numerous and widespread. Here are some, but certainly not all, of the many benefits (http:// www.nursingdegree.net/blog/24/77-surprising-health-benefits-of-yoga/):

1. Lower blood pressure
2. Lower pulse rate
3. Improved blood circulation

4. Lower respiratory rate
5. Greater cardiovascular endurance
6. Increased organ sensitivity
7. Improved gastrointestinal function
8. A more robust immune response
9. Higher tolerance to pain
10. Slows the aging process
11. Improves posture
12. Increases strength
13. Increases energy
14. Controls weight
15. Improves sleep
16. Improves balance
17. Increases body awareness
18. Improves sexual performance
19. Produces feelings of well-being
20. Reduces stress
21. Reduces anxiety
22. Reduces the possibility of depression
23. Increases self-control
24. Enhances the mind—body connection
25. Focuses concentration
26. Improves memory
27. Enhances social skills
28. Enhances serenity
29. Lowers cholesterol
30. Facilitates the flow of the lymphatic system
31. May lower blood glucose
32. Reduces sodium levels
33. Increases the production of red blood cells in the body
34. Reduces the risk of injury
35. Produces better muscle tone
36. Increases the range of joint range of motion
37. Enhances eye-hand coordination
38. Reduces the risk of heart disease

In addition to enthusiastic comments from many of his acquaintances, research addressing the numerous benefits of yoga deeply impressed John. Considering John's situation, regular yoga practice also appeared to help cancer patients. According to one site, it can enable cancer patients to "...gain strength, raise red blood cells, experience less nausea during chemotherapy, and have better overall well-being" (http://www.nursingdegree.net/blog/24/77-surprising-health-benefits-of-yoga/).

In its 2013 update on the benefits of yoga for cancer patients, the U.S. National Cancer Institute presented findings of various studies on the benefits of yoga for people undergoing cancer treatment. The topics covered included yoga breathing and the impact of chemotherapy, yoga and quality of life among breast cancer patients, yoga and cancer treatment fatigue, and yoga and the reduction of cancer treatment anxiety. (See http://cam.cancer.gov/yoga_breathing.html; http://cam.cancer.gov/breastcancer_yoga.html; http://cam.cancer.gov/annualreport/fy10/ar_yoga_fatigue.html; http://www.cancer.gov/cancertopics/pdq/supportivecare/adjustment/HealthProfessional/page1/AllPages#Section_518; http://nccam.nih.gov/video/yoga; http://nccam.nih.gov/health/yoga/introduction.htm).

Although the research results suggest some degree of caution is warranted in linking yoga practice to the enhancement of general health as well as the amelioration of side effects (both physical and psychological) of cancer treatment, there is very strong evidence that yoga is a good thing for anyone to do, especially if you are a cancer patient.

Despite its increased popularity, only a small percentage of adults engage in regular yoga practice. Even among those who report engaging in yoga, many of them label themselves beginners—people who have just started to do yoga or individuals who practice irregularly. The noncompetitive philosophy of yoga also appeals to many Americans. Although yoga can promote relaxation, time is a concern for many hardworking Americans and Europeans. If many Americans and Europeans, for example, don't have time to meditate for 15 to 20 minutes a day, how will they be able to spare 90 minutes to participate in a yoga class? There are other inhibiting factors. Older people may be intimidated by the relative youth of many yoga practitioners.

If a middle-aged man like John attends a yoga class, chances are he'll be the oldest person in the room and perhaps one of only a few males. Men may feel uncomfortable practicing something often perceived as a female activity. Some men may not like the fact that yoga poses can be similar to ballet or modern dance moves, which they see as the domain of females. Men who are not particularly limber may be embarrassed to demonstrate their lack of bodily grace in a room full of women.

JOHN DECIDES TO TAKE UP YOGA

John went to his first yoga flow class at the local YMCA. As expected, the auditorium-style room was filled with women—young, middle-aged, and older. He was one of three men in a class of 30 practitioners. The instructor was a middle-aged woman with a soft, soothing voice. She wore black tights and a sleeveless black training top. Most of the practitioners were dressed similarly and most carried the own mats.

John walked up to the instructor and introduced himself. "This is my first time."

"Wonderful." She pointed to a closet at the back of the room. "You should get yourself a mat and some blocks. Do what you can. Remember, the body knows best," she added cheerfully. "Remember that this is not a competition."

John got a mat and found a spot at the back of the classroom. The class started with breathing and stretching. He found the breathing exercises easy to do. As the class progressed, it became more difficult for him to keep up. Given his fatigue and bone aches, the forward bends, sun salutations, twists, and planks were quite challenging. Following the advice of the instructor, he did what his body would allow. If the poses hurt him, he would stop and put himself in a relaxing and soothing child's pose—on his knees with his forehead on the mat between his outstretched arms.

The practice made him realize the importance of accepting one's limitations, something he had not had to cope with prior to his cancer treatment. From the very first class, John enjoyed yoga. He didn't worry too much about his progress. He knew from his reading that in yoga, specific skills are less important than being present in the practice—feeling the body and focusing on breathing and thoughts. He especially enjoyed the relaxation pose, *Shavasana* or corpse pose. Lying on his back with his eyes closed, he let the soothing music enter his body. During this pose, he felt deep relaxation.

John could see why yoga was said to promote greater physical health and relaxation. Adding yoga to his schedule, he tried to attend a class three times a week. Because his meditation practice had become a morning routine at home, he felt he could take on another commitment, especially if it made him feel good. Like many other cancer patients, John began to see yoga practice as a kind of life-saver. No matter how weak he felt, he could always stretch and breathe. Furthermore, he always felt more relaxed after practicing a few minutes of yoga.

THE SUITABILITY OF YOGA

Like meditation, yoga is not for everyone. Not everybody can take on the noncompetitive, holistic aspects of yoga. For some men, the so-called "feminine" dimensions of yoga are a challenge that cannot be overcome. Indeed, some people would prefer to run or lift weights in the gym than move through an hour of yoga poses. Even so, a growing number of people are now taking up yoga, including, of course, cancer patients like John. Here are a few additional sources of information about the benefits of yoga for all practitioners, especially people undergoing treatment for cancer.

1. About yoga. Asheville Yoga Center website. Accessed at http://www. youryoga.com/ayc/~info.html on May 23, 2008.
2. Bower, JE, Woolery, A, Sternlieb, B, Garet, D. Yoga for cancer patients and survivors. *Cancer Control.* 2005; 12:165-171.
3. Cohen L, Warneke C, Fouladi RT, Rodriguez MA, Chaoul-Reich A. Psychological adjustment and sleep quality in a randomized trial of

the effects of a Tibetan yoga intervention in patients with lymphoma. *Cancer.* 2004; 100:2253-2260.

4. McDonald A, Burjan E, Martin S. Yoga for patients and careers in a palliative day care setting. *Int J Palliat Nurs.* 2006; 12:519-523.

5. Moadel AB, Shah C, Wylie-Rosett J, et al. Randomized controlled trial of yoga among a multiethnic sample of breast cancer patients: effects on quality of life. *J Clin Oncol.* 2007; 25:4387-4395.

6. National Institutes of Health. *Alternative Medicine: Expanding Medical Horizons: A Report to the National Institutes of Health on Alternative Medical Systems and Practices in the United States.* Washington, DC: US Government Printing Office; 1994. NIH publication 94-066.

7. Taylor, E. Yoga and meditation. *Altern Ther Health Med.*1995; 1:77-78.

11 MASSAGE AND REFLEXOLOGY

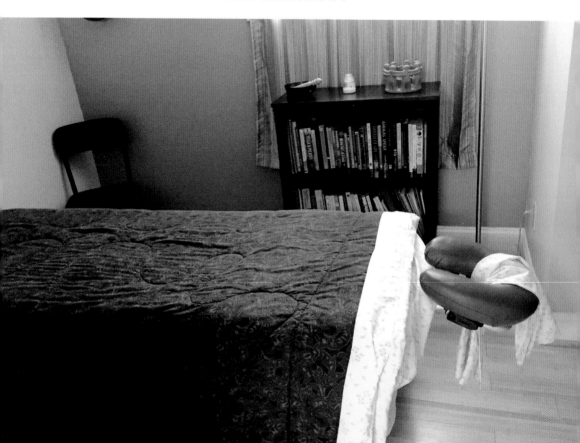

Like other cancer patients, John's life had become largely focused on ways to manage his illness and promote his well-being. He was amazed when he remembered that he had given very little thought to his health before cancer. He had never had to pay much attention to what he needed to do to stay energetic, or even just to make it through his day. His treatment was grueling. The cumulative effects of chemotherapy depleted his energy. As weeks turned into months, John found that his struggle to maintain his routine became more and more difficult.

At this point John was open to every possibility that might lead to well-being. He meditated most mornings for 20 minutes, and he did yoga three times a week. He continued his daily walks, although they were not as long as they had been. He and Beth still socialized with family and friends, although not as frequently. The five-hour treatment sessions, once every three weeks, took a toll on his body.

Understanding John's difficulties, Beth gave John a gift certificate for a therapeutic massage. John had had a massage for relaxation a few times in his life. Now he needed massage to help with his aches and pains. As treatment continued, John found that his aches and pains and the degree of fatigue had increased. The side effects, which were most intense for the first week after treatment, now lingered for ten days to two weeks after treatment. Just when he began to feel relatively "normal," it would be time for another round of chemotherapy.

John became friendly with his fellow patients and his nurses. Although it may seem odd, John even looked forward to seeing them. Even so, the prospect of another five-hour drip of toxic medicine into his bloodstream provoked considerable anxiety. Additionally, it was becoming increasingly difficult to find a vein that had not been overused. Despite this litany of troubles, John continued to count his blessings. He realized that despite his suffering, he was still lucky. He had not lost his hair. He could taste his food and had not suffered from mouth sores. His weight had stabilized. Unlike many of his fellow patients, he hadn't experienced ongoing nausea, and his white and red blood cell counts had remained within normal ranges. John's oncologist was hopeful and positive.

"Each person responds differently to treatment," he explained. "You began your treatment in good physical shape. You jogged, hiked, biked, and worked out. That always helps."

"No matter how fit you are," Beth said when John talked with her about his growing aches and pains, "The impact of chemo is devastating. I think you've fared well because you took steps to reduce the impact of the side effects. You continued to exercise. You took up meditation and began to practice yoga—all of which have helped you. The meditation calms your mind and the yoga stretches and tones your body."

John realized that the cancer experience had actually broadened his awareness of life. It had compelled him to try new wellness activities that he might have otherwise avoided—yoga and meditation. It had made him appreciate his health, his good days, and his relationships.

He now often combined yoga and meditation, practicing yoga several times a week and finishing each session with 15 minutes of meditation. Over time, the effects of chemotherapy compelled John to reduce the level of his yoga practice, but he found that the balance between yoga and meditation continued to be effective for him. These activities made him more flexible.

Despite these ongoing wellness activities, John's fatigue and bone pain continued. He also continued to feel stressed about how illness would affect his future. A positive CT scan report indicated that John's abdominal tumor had shrunk by 50 percent. Such good news, however, did not make his anxious feelings of uncertainty dissipate, which prompted John to search for new methods that might ease some of his pain and anxiety.

John's doctor and his friendly and helpful oncology nurse both suggested he try getting a massage.

"The research is inconclusive, but most studies suggest that massage and reflexology relieve pain and lower blood pressure. Most patients report that they make you incredibly relaxed and give you a greater sense of well-being," his oncology nurse told him. She recounted stories of former patients who had tried both massage and reflexology. "They found it very beneficial."

John went home to conduct background research on the potential benefits of massage.

SOME FUNDAMENTALS OF MASSAGE AND REFLEXOLOGY

Just as meditation and yoga have become more commonly practiced in Europe and North America, so too have massage and reflexology. In past generations, massage was seen in two ways: (1) a way that wealthy people could relax from the hectic pace of their business or social schedules; or (2) a therapeutic exercise for athletes who needed to soothe sore muscles or recover from minor injuries. In the latter case, you might go to the gym, work out for one hour, and retire to the locker room where an attendant masseuse would give you a rubdown.

Massage and reflexology are associated with the notion of wellness, a program of activities that direct people into arenas of well-being. As such, therapeutic massage and reflexology have become a one-billion-dollar industry in the U.S., according to Dr. Mark Rapaport, chairman of the department of psychiatry and behavioral neurosciences at Cedars-Sinai Medical Center in Los Angeles. Rapaport has conducted studies on the physical and emotion ramifications of massage. In his study, he considered how massage affected the conditions of 53 subjects and found that light touch Swedish massage sessions reduced stress hormones and increased white blood cell counts, which suggested an increased robustness of the immune system (http://www.oprah.com/health/The-Health-Benefits-of-Massage).

The Mayo Clinic website mentions the four most common forms of massage.

+ **Swedish massage.** This is a gentle form of massage that uses long strokes, kneading, deep circular movements, vibration, and tapping to help relax and energize you.

+ **Deep massage.** This massage technique uses slower, more forceful strokes to target the deeper layers of muscle and connective tissue and is commonly used to help with muscle damage from injuries.
+ **Sports massage.** This is similar to Swedish massage, but it's geared toward people involved in sport activities to help prevent or treat injuries.
+ **Trigger point massage.** This massage focuses on areas of tight muscle fibers that can form in your muscles after injuries or overuse.

SOME OF THE POTENTIAL BENEFITS OF MASSAGE INCLUDE:

+ Reduce anxiety
+ Aid digestive disorders
+ Soothe the pain of fibromyalgia
+ Ease headaches
+ Reduce insomnia related to stress
+ Reduce the effects of myofascial pain syndrome
+ Ease paresthesia and nerve pain
+ Aid the healing of soft tissue strains or injuries
+ Reduce the severity of sports injuries
+ Reduce temporomandibular joint pain (http://www.mayoclinic.org/healthy-living/stress-management/in-depth/massage/art-20045743)

MASSAGE DURING CANCER TREATMENT

Major centers for cancer treatment recommend therapeutic massage as a way of dealing with both the emotional and physical side effects of chemotherapy and radiation treatments. In a 2013 study, Karagozuglu and Kahve found that back massage reduced the levels of stress and fatigue that most patients experience after chemotherapy treatments ("Effects of back massage on chemotherapy-related fatigue and anxiety: supportive care and therapeutic touch in cancer nursing." *Applied Nursing Research* 26(4): 210-217).

The American Cancer Society draws the following conclusion on the benefits of massages for cancer patients. They write:

> While massage appears promising for symptom management and improving quality of life, available scientific evidence does not support claims that massage slows or reverses the growth or spread of cancer. A growing number of health care professionals recognize massage as a useful addition to conventional medical treatment. In a 1999 publication, the National Cancer Institute found that about half of their cancer centers offered massage as an adjunctive therapy to cancer treatment. Some studies of massage for cancer patients suggest that it can decrease stress, anxiety, depression, pain, and fatigue. These potential benefits hold great promise for people who have cancer, who often must deal with the stresses of a serious illness in addition to unpleasant side effects of conventional medical treatment. While some evidence from research studies with cancer patients supports the use of massage for short-term symptom relief, additional research is needed to find out if there are measurable, long-term physical or psychological benefits.
>
> Meanwhile, most patients do indeed seem to feel better after massage, which may result in substantial relief. A 2005 review of research reported that massage therapy has been shown to reduce pain and anxiety in randomized controlled trials. Large, well-controlled studies are still needed to determine the long-term health benefits of massage (http://www.cancer.org/treatment/treatmentsandsideeffects/complementaryandalternativemedicine/manualhealingandphysicaltouch/massage).

REFLEXOLOGY

Massage may make people uncomfortable. Some people may not want strangers to touch them. There are many alternatives to lying under a sheet unclothed on a massage table. Massage chairs are effective and enable the recipients to remain fully clothed. There are also therapeutic partial massages, such as reflexology. Although the claims about reflexology's impact on specific parts of the body still trigger scientific debate, many people say that foot massage, during which you sit on a recliner or lay fully clothed on a massage table while the therapist rubs your feet, is deeply relaxing and therefore highly therapeutic for a wide range of conditions, including cancer. For cancer patients, some studies suggest that regular reflexology sessions can reduce stress, relieve pain, and promote a feeling of well-being. Studies in the UK have found that cancer patients consider reflexology a popular form of alternative treatment (http://www.cancer.org/treatment/treatmentsandsideeffects/complementaryandalternativemedicine/manualhealingandphysicaltouch/massage).

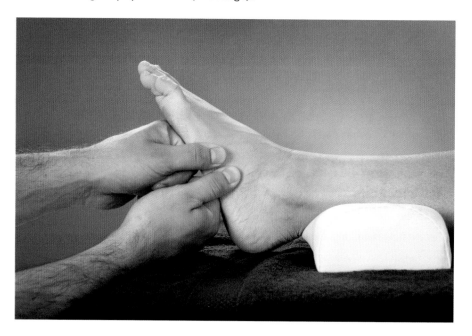

JOHN'S REFLEXOLOGY EXPERIENCE

Convinced of the possible benefits of massage and reflexology and able to afford these treatments, John decided to start with reflexology. On the day of his appointment, he drove a few blocks to a local wellness clinic. He entered a soothing dark space infused with incense. Just inside the door, there was fountain that made John think of the water gushing over the stones of a creek, a place where he and his childhood friends liked to play.

The receptionist greeted him pleasantly and gave him some patient information forms to fill out. "Fill those out, and I'll tell Ann that you're here."

John filled out the forms and Ann, a tall, middle-aged woman with blond hair and a pleasant smile, introduced herself to him.

"John, you look nervous," Anne said. "Don't be. I've been doing body work for 25 years."

"Okay."

They entered a small, dimly lit room. Soft, relaxing music played in the background. Ann pointed to a chair in the corner.

"Take off your shoes and socks and roll up your pants legs. I'll be right back."

John did as he was instructed and remained on the chair. A fountain pushed water over rocks awash in dim purple light.

Anne re-entered the room with a tub of what seemed like scented water. "I'll wash your feet first. The water is warm. It should relax you."

Anne rubbed both of his feet, which did put him at ease.

"Close your eyes and try to let go of all the stress in your body."

Ann asked him to get up on the massage bed and lay down on his back. She put a pillow under his head and a bolster under his knees. She positioned herself in front of his bare feet at the head of the massage bed.

She put her warm hands on his feet, gently moving them to a 45-degree angle. "Take three deep breaths, John."

Then she began to work on his feet, first pushing on the toes and pad of his left foot and then doing the same on his right foot. Then she slowly moved down to the middle of his feet and put gentle pressure on his arches. Eventually she worked down to his heels and rubbed his ankles and calves. Toward the end, she applied massage oil to his feet and worked her hands over his toes, foot pads, and arches.

John experienced almost immediate relaxation. His deeply relaxed state allowed his mind to take him to new places, some of which he had visited, some of which he had only imagined. He imagined himself relaxing in cool, soothing forests. He imagined the redwood forests along the California coast that he had visited as a young man. He pictured himself on a sunny beach. During the treatment, he felt that he was in an in-between state, somewhere between sleep and consciousness. The images in his mind were alternately hazy and clear.

After what seemed like a very short amount of time, he heard Anne's voice ask him to take a deep breath. She had again moved his feet to an angle. He took three deep breaths and slowly opened his eyes.

"Take your time, John. I'll see you at the front desk," Anne said.

John was amazed that 45 minutes had passed so quickly. He felt strong as well as peaceful. Unlike his other experiments, like yoga and meditation (the benefits of which had taken time to develop), the positive effects of reflexology seemed immediate.

As he slowly rolled down the legs of his jeans and put on his shoes and socks, John felt a sense of peace, even contentment—something he had been missing for months. He knew that he would continue reflexology sessions during and after the conclusion of his cancer treatments. He was hooked.

Anne stood by the desk and gave John a hug. "Well?"

"It was amazing," he said. "I'll definitely be back." As he was leaving, John made a new appointment.

Not everyone will respond positively to reflexology—or massage—as did John.

According to the results of ongoing research, reflexology and massage are not cures for cancer, but they seem to be able to alleviate the stresses and strains that accompany cancer treatment and give patients a measure of well-being—always a good thing—as they confront the ongoing challenges of climbing the mountain. Here is a small sampling of resources on the benefits that massage (and reflexology) can bring to cancer patients.

RESOURCES ON MASSAGE (AND REFLEXOLOGY) AND CANCER

1. American Cancer Society. Massage. http://www. cancer.org/treatment/treatmentsandsideeffects/ complementaryandalternativemedicine/ manualhealingandphysicaltouch/massage.
2. Walton, Tracy. 2014. *Massage Therapy, Oncology Massage Guidelines*. http://tracywalton.com/
3. Walton, Tracy. 2011. *Medical Conditions and Massage Therapy: A Decision-Tree Approach*. Boston: Philadelphia, PA: Lippincott Williams & Wilkins
4. Wong, Kathy. 2014. *4 Benefits of Massage for People with Cancer*. Altmedicine, About Heath. http://altmedicine.about.com/od/cance1/a/massage_cancer.htm
5. MacDonald, Gayle 2003. *Cancer, Radiation and Massage: The Benefits and Cautions*. Massage Therapy.com http://www. massagetherapy.com/articles/index.php/article_id/184/Cancer-Radiation-and-Massage
6. Cancer Council. 2014. *The Benefits of Massage to Cancer Patients*. http://www.cancercouncil.com.au/17958/b1000/massage-and-cancer-42/massage-and-cancer-benefits-of-touch/
7. Fellowes D, Barnes K, Wilkinson SSM. 2008. Aromatherapy and massage for symptoms relief in patients with cancer. *Cochrane Database of Systematic Reviews 4*.
8. Cassileth BR, Vickers AJ. Massage therapy for symptom control: outcome study at a major cancer centre. *J Pain Symptom Manage 2004 Sep; 28 (3): 244–9*.

9. Stringer J et al. 2008 Massage in patients undergoing intensive chemotherapy reduces serum cortisol and prolactin. *Psycho-Oncology* 2008 17 (10): 1024–31.
10. Sturgeon M, Wetta-Hall R, Hart T, Good M, Dakhil S. 2009. Effects of therapeutic massage on the quality of life among patients with breast cancer during treatment. *Journal of Alternative and Complementary Medicine* 15(4):373-80.

12 SOCIAL SUPPORT

No one should have to confront cancer alone. Social science research has long suggested that people who are seriously challenged by illness or a sudden life transition seem to respond creatively and more robustly to the challenges of social and personal change if they have some form of social support. Social support is usually defined as the presence of family, friends, colleagues, and social institutions (churches, synagogues, mosques, and organizations, such as

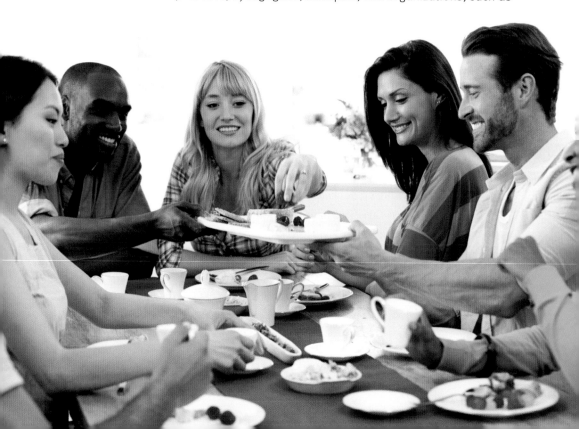

Kiwanis or Rotary clubs). Satisfying social support provides resources that reduce feelings of isolation and perceptions of helplessness. It is the quality rather than the quantity of support that is important. One or two close friends can be sufficient support for one person. Additional relationships might be stressful for some people. Another person might require a larger circle of friends and family to feel a sense of satisfaction. Studies have found that the presence of satisfying networks of social support appears to have positive and significant effects for people who must follow cancer's path.

More general social support appears to benefit people, including cancer patients, in a number of significant ways. It improves the overall quality of life. It also reduces:

+ Anxiety and stress
+ Emotional distress and depression
+ Fatigue
+ The experience of pain

SOCIAL SUPPORT IMPROVES:

+ Mood
+ Self-image
+ Ability to cope with stress
+ Sexual function and enjoyment
+ Feelings of control

http://ww5.komen.org/BreastCancer/BenefitsofSocialSupport.html

CANCER AND RELATIONSHIPS

John had already been briefly introduced to a cancer support group and found it helpful. When confronted with his illness, John's relationships with Beth, his other family members, and his colleagues became more precious to him. His confrontation with mortality had enriched his relationship with Beth. He understood how difficult it was for her to be supportive during his cancer treatment. He was grateful for the continuous support of his friends. He realized that it was difficult for them to know what to say to him, how much help to offer, when to visit, and when to leave John alone.

CAREGIVING STRESS

Beth, who was John's primary support person, had a particularly difficult time managing her own life as a caregiver. Like millions of other Americans and Europeans, Beth found caregiving exceedingly stressful. Caregiving is usually an unpaid role that a spouse, partner, family member, or friend takes on to help someone in need. It involves providing assistance with instrumental as well as emotional needs.

HERE IS A COMPILATION OF STATISTICS ABOUT CAREGIVERS:

- 65.7 million caregivers make up 29% of the U.S. adult population, providing care to someone who is ill, disabled or aged.
  [The National Alliance for Caregiving and AARP (2009), Caregiving in the U.S. National Alliance for Caregiving. Washington, DC.] - **Updated: November 2012**

- 52 million caregivers provide care to adults (aged 18+) with a disability or illness.
  [Coughlin, J., (2010). Estimating the Impact of Caregiving and Employment on Well-Being: Outcomes & Insights in Health Management, Vol. 2; Issue 1] - **Updated: November 2012**

- 43.5 million of adult family caregivers care for someone 50+ years of age, and 14.9 million care for someone who has Alzheimer's disease or other dementia.
  [Alzheimer's Association, 2011 Alzheimer's Disease Facts and Figures, Alzheimer's and Dementia, Vol.7, Issue 2.] - **Updated: November 2012**

- Caregiver services were valued at $450 billion per year in 2009—up from $375 billion in year 2007.
  [Valuing the Invaluable: 2011 Update, The Economic Value of Family Caregiving. AARP Public Policy Institute.] - **Updated: November 2012**

- The value of unpaid family caregivers will likely continue to be the largest source of long-term care services in the U.S., and the aging population (65+) will more than double between the years 2000 and 2030, increasing to 71.5 million from 35.1 million in 2000.
  [Coughlin, J., (2010). Estimating the Impact of Caregiving and Employment on Well-Being: Outcomes & Insights in Health Management, Vol. 2; Issue 1] - **Updated: November 2012**

https://www.caregiver.org/selected-caregiver-statistics

Like Beth, the majority of caregivers are women. Caregiving demands time and effort. Even so, most caregivers have full-time jobs as well as other social responsibilities, which make caregiving even more difficult. In addition, concern about a loved one's suffering further increases caregiving stress. Studies have shown that there are significant health risks linked to providing long-term care. Many caregivers experience anxiety and depression (National Alliance for Caregiving in collaboration with AARP, 2009).

Caregivers also need support. Studies have found that caregivers respond favorably to a variety of interventions, including mindfulness training, individual therapy, technological support, support groups, and the use of home health care providers, as well as additional help with errands and transportation that family and friends can provide. Caregivers like Beth, who was in her forties and who is familiar with Internet research, have been found to benefit considerably from online informational and emotional support.

Guilt over caregiving stress is also a source of concern for caregivers. After all, they are not the ones who need care. Sharing feelings, reading information on caregiving, and seeking support from other caregivers can be helpful. For her part, Beth joined an online caregiving support group in which she could freely express her concerns and share her feelings.

Support groups, including online support groups, are helpful for caregivers. Groups present information, teach coping skills, and provide a place to share feelings. There are many different types of support groups available for caregivers. In the U.S. alone, 500,000 self-help groups exist, with as many as 15 million people participating at some point in their lives (Work Group for Community Health and Development, 2013). Support groups reduce the risk of social isolation.

JOHN'S SUPPORT GROUP

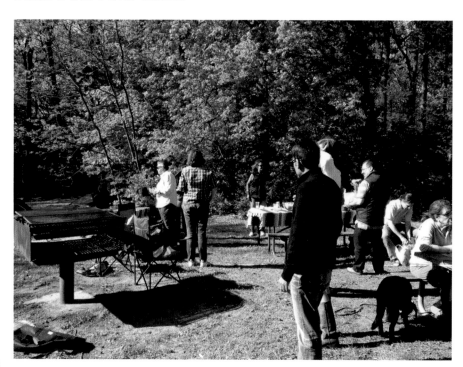

As mentioned previously, John also attended a support group. Like other cancer patients, he wanted to experience the feeling of camaraderie that develops among others who are undergoing a similar experience. Despite his substantial network of support, John felt lonely at times. His illness gave him a sense of alienation. He sensed that none of his friends, family, or colleagues could really understand what he was going through. How could they know what it was like to hear the phrase: "I'm sorry, John, but I'm afraid you have cancer?" How could they know what it was like to sit in a treatment chair for five hours as chemotherapy medicines dripped into his bloodstream? How could they know what it was like to sit by the phone, waiting for a CT scan report that could bring a verdict of life or death?

His doctor and his nurses listened to John talk about his feelings, something he would not have done prior to his illness.

"Your loneliness is not unusual, John," his oncology nurse stated. "Many patients experience periods of loneliness and disconnection."

"But there are people around. I'm not alone. I can freely express my concerns with my loved ones, friends, and colleagues. I just don't understand why that's not enough for me."

"Sometimes you can feel lonely in a crowd, John. Maybe what's really going on is that people who haven't shared your cancer experience cannot understand the depth of your fear and uncertainty."

"Yes. I feel like other patients know what I know—about cancer, about life. And you know what? I feel that common understanding almost instantaneously—a silent dialogue."

The nurse nodded. "That's why we encourage our patients to participate in support groups. Are you doing that? Not everyone likes them, but they seem to make people feel less isolated. We have a support group of people who have had your type of cancer. They meet twice a month on Wednesdays at the Unitarian Church. Here's a brochure and the address of the organizer. Why not call her and attend the next meeting? I think it's next week."

With some hesitation, John made the phone call. Beth wanted to go with him, but John felt that it would be better to go alone. He arrived at the Unitarian Church and was greeted by a friendly-looking older woman, Susan, who was a social worker, a fellow cancer patient, and the support group's organizer.

"Hi, John. Welcome." She gave him a nametag to wear. "Still in treatment?" she asked.

"Yes. It's been five months."

"And you still have your hair?" she asked playfully.

John blushed. "Some of it."

"We think it's important to joke about these experiences, if possible. It makes it easier to talk about them. There's too much seriousness in our world, don't you think?"

"Yes, I agree."

"Follow me and I'll introduce you." John entered a softly lit conference room, where sofas and chairs had been positioned in a circle around a long coffee table on which someone had arranged an assortment of bread, hummus, olives, cheese, and cookies. The strong aroma of coffee wafted into the room. Susan turned toward John. "At least you won't leave here feeling hungry."

Susan introduced John to the other participants. Like John, some of the people were in the middle of treatment. A few of them had completed initial treatment only to return months or years later for additional interventions because the cancer had returned. Others had been "cancer free" for longer periods of time. One man he met had been "cancer free" for 15 years.

"If you've been cancer free for 15 years, why are you here?"

He smiled. "It can come back at any time, John. Besides, these people understand me in ways that no one else can."

After some eating and chatting, Susan facilitated the group discussion, asking each of the 12 participants to share something that was bothering them. John found some of the stories illuminating and reassuring. Before his illness he would not have had time for such storytelling. But cancer had transformed his sensibilities. He found himself more open and accepting. When it was his turn, he talked hesitantly about his increasing feelings of isolation. Everyone nodded. They knew what he was experiencing, which made him feel much less isolated in the world. When the meeting ended, Susan asked him if he would be back.

"I liked the session, but talking about my feelings with strangers is new to me. It's a bit unsettling."

"But they're strangers who have been through what you've been through."

"True. That's important and helpful."

"You can also try to get support by joining an online discussion group. There's a good one for lymphoma patients." She wrote down the web address of the site. "Go online and take part in the electronic discussion. It has the advantage of being available all the time."

John went to a few more support group meetings at the Unitarian Church, but he found the support group activity on social media to be more convenient and almost as helpful. As John plodded through his treatment, he was able to go online at his convenience, read about the concerns of fellow patients, and express his own feelings. He found the participation and support emotionally helpful.

CANCER SUPPORT GROUPS

Many cancer treatment centers encourage patients to participate in support groups, which exist for every imaginable emotional and physical disorder, including, of course, support groups for every kind of cancer. If the local cancer treatment center doesn't sponsor support groups, most communities have wellness centers at which various kinds of support groups meet. Although the primary model for the support group involves face-to-face contact, a growing number of cancer patients are using forms of social media: virtual support groups that, in addition to providing an online forum for discussion of patient concerns, regularly share the results of the latest research on the biology of cancer as well as the outcomes of clinical trials. These sites can be treasure troves of general and specific information on cancer.

Writers for the American Cancer Society (ACS) provide a very concise description of support groups, which constitute a key component of the ACS website.

> Many different kinds of support groups are available, and they vary in their structure and activities. Some are time-limited, while others are ongoing. Some support groups are made up of people with the same type of cancer, while others include people who are having the same kind of treatment. Support groups are available for patients, family members, and other caregivers of people who have cancer, and even children with cancer in the family. The format of different groups varies from lectures and discussions to exploration and expression of feelings. Behavioral training can involve muscle relaxation or meditation to reduce stress and cope with the effects of chemotherapy or radiation therapy. Topics addressed in support groups are those of concern to the members and those the group leader thinks are important. (http://www.cancer.org/treatment/treatmentsandsideeffects/ complementaryandalternativemedicine/mindbodyandspirit/support-groups-cam)

As we have indicated, there are literally hundreds of social media websites devoted to social support. Virtual support groups are especially attractive to patients who don't particularly care for face-to-face group activities. Some people just don't want to join a group and share a potentially embarrassing illness narrative with strangers.

Whether they involve face-to face encounters or conversations through social media, the reason for the breadth and depth of cancer support groups is clear. Many cancer patients may not even be aware of the research that suggests that participation in any kind of support group is highly beneficial. Some other patients may believe, though the results of clinical research on whether social support extends survival are far from conclusive, that joining a support group may extend their lives or even cure their cancer (http://www.cancer.org/treatment/treatmentsandsideeffects/complementaryandalternativemedicine/mindbodyandspirit/support-groups-cam).

From a more anthropological perspective, support groups tend to extend the feeling of the aforementioned communitas beyond the confines of the treatment room in which many cancer patients, as reported in Chapter 7, feel a silent and powerful sense of camaraderie—a feeling shared only by those who have directly experienced the existential concerns and questions caused by cancer. In a sense, support group participation underscores and strengthens that silent bond. From the patient's perspective, people who share their deeply personal experiences in support groups are fellow travelers on the path that takes you higher and higher up on the mountain—a trail on which you continuously need a "little help from your friends."

TREATMENT AND CHANGES IN RELATIONSHIPS

John's treatment compelled him to slow down and relax. As a result, he also had more time to talk with Beth and be with his friends and extended family. He was able to accommodate their schedules and spend more quality time with them. As a result of his illness, he felt that he had learned to appreciate more fully the people in his life. John's networks of relations constituted a model for positive social support, which, as stated, can have many positive benefits for cancer patients.

The overall social environment seems to play a strong role in the survival rate of cancer patients. Satisfying social support can help alleviate the negative effects of stress associated with cancer; it can also help cancer patients feel less isolated and stigmatized. Studies have found that cancer patients with satisfying social support have greater survival rates. In one study, women who were socially isolated were 34 percent more likely to die from breast cancer than women who were socially integrated. The same study found that satisfying family relationships, community ties, and religious support were critical for survival (http://www.medicinenet.com/script/main/art.asp?articlekey=165120).

People clearly need other people to survive, especially during difficult periods. We have a need to connect with others. Historically, social connections have been linked to survival in hostile environments. Relationships exist within a social framework. They are in a continuous state of flux. As you age, your life circumstances change. If you become ill, your relationships also change.

John's illness had changed the texture of his relationships. It had made him appreciate the people in his life. It had brought him closer to Beth. Even so, his illness made him feel socially isolated. Studies have shown that when cancer patients are diagnosed, they may experience feelings of guilt and blame, a loss of control, avoidance, anger, sorrow, withdrawal, and loneliness and isolation. These feelings can have a significant, negative impact on a cancer patient's family and friends. If cancer patients enter remission, family and friends may be so relieved that they are ready to just move on, whereas the patients are still struggling with life in remission. They know that they will never go back to life before cancer, something that may be difficult for their loved ones to understand.

THE PHYSICAL AND EMOTIONAL BENEFITS OF SOCIAL SUPPORT

In 2012, Larry Berkelhammer, an expert on mindfulness and immune response, reported in a blog post that:

> In a substantial study of three thousand breast cancer patients, all of whom were nurses, completed in 2006, researchers found that women without close friends had a mortality rate four times that of women with a close circle of friends.

In another study of 514 women, 239 were diagnosed with breast cancer. One of the results of this study was that those with the least social support were nine times as likely to develop cancer following a stressful life event. In fact, most psycho-oncology studies have found a positive correlation between survival times after cancer diagnosis and the amount and quality of social support. (http://www.larryberkelhammer.com/cancer/cancer-and-social-support#)

In the same blog post, Berkelhammer wrote about the epidemiological research of Elizabeth Maunsell, who had asked 244 breast cancer patients how many people they had confided to during a three-month period following cancer surgery. Here are the results:

+ The seven-year survival rate for the patients who had not confided in anyone during that three-month post-surgery period was 56 percent.
+ The survival rate for those who had confided in one person was 66 percent.
+ Those who had confided in two or more people had a 76 percent survival rate. (http://www.larryberkelhammer.com/cancer/cancer-and-social-support#)

Social support can take many forms. Marriage is a major source of social support. But forging some other kinds of social relationships can also can also help people respond well to serious illnesses like cancer. In the absence of or in addition to the support of family, friends, and organizations, individuals can also seek out patient advocates (described in Chapter 2). Beyond family, friends, and organizational and advocate support, many cancer patients attempt to find support from those who have experienced similar trauma through a support group.

SUPPORT AND THE CANCER EXPERIENCE

Each person's illness is unique, but concerns about pain, nausea, hair loss, and our end-of-life fears can be shared with other patients. John was lucky. He had a supportive partner, family members, and a few close friends. He was able to satisfy some of his emotional needs by talking with fellow patients during treatment sessions and in support groups. Regardless of the degree of support, however, there is no escape from some measure of loneliness, the rate of which, according to Jessica Olien's 2013 article in *Slate,* has doubled during the last 20 years (http://www.slate.com/articles/health_and_science/medical_examiner/2013/08/dangers_of_loneliness_social_isolation_is_deadlier_than_obesity.html). Unfortunately, many cancer patients do not have the social support that John had.

As we've stated, there is a substantial literature on all aspects of social support. Here we provide some major websites that provide useful information on and forums for social support. There is also a list of some of the major studies that underscore the emotional and potential physical benefits of social support and a list of sites for general information on the cancer experience.

SOME MAJOR STUDIES ON SOCIAL SUPPORT

1. Ikeda A1, Kawachi I, Iso H, Iwasaki M, Inoue M, Tsugane S. 2013. Social support and cancer incidence and mortality: the JPHC study cohort II.
    Cancer Causes Control. 2013 May;24(5):847-60. doi: 10.1007/s10552-013-0147-7. Epub Apr 3.
2. Candyce H. Kroenke, Laura D. Kubzansky, Eva S. Schernhammer, Michelle D. Holmes and Ichiro Kawachi. 2006. Social Networks, Social Support, and Survival After Breast Cancer Diagnosis. *JournaRel of Clinical Oncology 24*(7): 1105-1111.
3. Pennebaker, J. (1990). *Opening Up: The Healing Power of Confiding in Others.* New York: Morrow.
4. Helgelston, Vicki, and Sheldon Cohen 1996. Social Support and Adjustment to Cancer. Reconciling Decescritive, Correlative and Intervention Research. *Health Psychology 15*(2): 135-148.

A SAMPLE OF BOOKS ON CANCER—AND SOCIAL SUPPORT

1.   The American Cancer society publishes a series of books on cancer and emotional support. These can be found at the ACS online bookstores and range from stories of family stress and support to how to adjust social support in families in which a child is suffering from cancer. http://www.cancer.org/cancer/bookstore/emotional-support-books.

2.   Kneece, Judy 2012. *Breast Cancer Treatment Handbook: Understanding the Disease, Treatments, Emotions, and Recovery from Breast Cancer.* Charleston, SC: Educare.

3.   Barraclaugh, Jennifer 1998. *Cancer and Emotion: A Practical Guide to Psycho-Oncology.* New York: John Wiley and Sons.

4.   Alsop, Stuart. 1973. *Stay of Execution.* Philadelphia: Lippincott.

5.   Goodreads. *Memoirs by People with Cancer.* http://www.goodreads.com/list/show/42705.Memoirs_by_people_with_cancer

MAJOR RESOURCES FOR CANCER AND SOCIAL SUPPORT (GO TO THE SITE AND CLICK ON SUPPORT OR SUPPORT GROUPS)

1.   American Cancer Society. http://www.cancer.org/treatment/treatmentsandsideeffects/complementaryandalternativemedicine/mindbodyandspirit/support-groups-cam.

2.   American Council on Cancer Research. How to Find a Support Group. http://www.aacr.org/AdvocacyPolicy/SurvivorPatientAdvocacy/PAGES/HOW-TO-FIND-A-SUPPORT-GROUP.ASPX#.VKwyAidO2T8.

3.   Association of Cancer Online Resources. http://acor.org/

4.   American Lung Association. http://www.lung.org/lung-disease/lung-cancer/

5.   The Livestrong Foundation. http://www.livestrong.org/

6.   National Cancer Institute. http://www.cancer.gov/

7.   The Skin Cancer Foundation. http://www.skincancer.org/

8.   The Prostate Cancer Foundation. http://www.pcf.org/site/c.leJRIROrEpH/b.5699537/k.BEF4/Home.htm

9. Lymphoma Research Foundation. http://www.lymphoma.org/site/pp. asp?c=bkLTKaOQLmK8E&b=6296735

10. National Breast Cancer Foundation. http://www. nationalbreastcancer.org/breast-cancer-support.

11. National Cancer Institute (NCI) at The National Institutes of Health. (Find an NCI designated Cancer Center. http://www.cancer.gov/ researchandfunding/extramural/cancercenters/find-a-cancer-center

MAJOR ONLINE SUPPORT AND DISCUSSION GROUPS

1. The Wellness Community. Online Cancer Support. http://www. cancersupportcommunity.org/MainMenu/Cancer-Support/Online-Support-Groups.html

2. American Cancer Society. Cancer Survivors Network. http://csn. cancer.org/forum.

3. Cancercare: Counseling, Support Groups, Education, Financial Assistance. http://www.cancercare.org/support_groups.

4. Breastcancer.org. Community. http://www.breastcancer.org/ community.

5. The Carcinoid Cancer Foundation. http://www.carcinoid.org/content/ online-support-and-discussion-groups.

6. Lymphomation.org. Patients Against Lymphoma. http://www. lymphomation.org/support-groups.htm

7. Lymphoma.com. Lymphoma support and help forums http://forums. lymphoma.com/

Exploration of any of these sites may provide important information that will help cancer patients make informed decisions about standard as well as complementary treatments. Participation in online discussions about cancer diagnosis, treatment, and other experiences may decrease the sense of isolation that many cancer patients confront during their particular experience.

13 POST-TREATMENT BLUES

Like many cancer patients, John had come to feel comfortable during treatment sessions, which transpired once every three weeks. Treatment forced him to slow down. He continued to work but on a part-time basis. He had fewer client meetings to attend, less research to conduct, and no late-night, last-minute contract writing. His colleagues wanted him to take a paid leave of absence, but because he felt it was important for him to keep his life as "normal" as possible, he continued to work as much as he could. By slowing down, John had time to drive to state parks, where he would take trails that led through the forests and hills of his community. Beth accompanied him whenever she could. These walks brought John and Beth closer together.

The treatment-induced slower lifestyle also got John in the gym more regularly. The side effects from chemotherapy, of course, imposed limitations, but activity made John feel good. Beth also urged him to continue with his massages to reduce the physical and psychological impact of chemotherapy treatments.

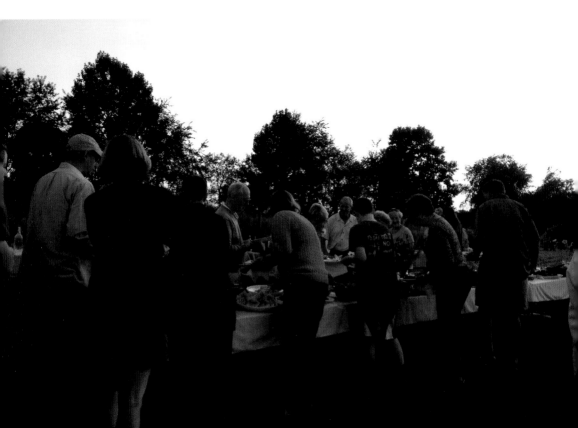

Cancer treatment had in some ways unexpectedly brought John's life into balance. He came to appreciate "the little things." His slow walks through the forest heightened his senses. He now noticed smells and sounds that he had overlooked. He found himself to be more patient. Despite the uncertainty of his future, treatment made John feel comfortable with himself.

At his last treatment session, John felt a sense of regret. He was elated that this phase of his cancer experience was now complete, but he did not know what to expect in the future. Soon after the end of his treatment, John's colleagues organized a party to celebrate. Everyone was there—senior partners, junior partners, associates, staff, and families. John's colleagues feted him like a conquering hero. They took turns speaking about John's courage and character.

"He never gave up."

"He never complained."

"John is a warrior—a survivor."

John didn't know how to respond to these comments. He appreciated them, but he didn't feel like he had conquered anything. He didn't feel brave or heroic. At that moment he wondered if he would able to return to his previous life, as if nothing had changed. John felt that no one at the party understood what he had been through. He felt isolated and sad.

DEPRESSION FOLLOWING TREATMENT

Most cancer patients get the blues. When we hear the words, "I'm sorry, but you have cancer," the first question you ask is: "What's the prognosis?"

" Well, you have a 50/50 chance of survival."

When we hear those odds, to quote the great blues guitarist, Buddy Guy, we think, "You damn right I got the blues. From my head right down to my shoes."

We all get the blues. It is an integral part of the human experience. When cancer patients begin their long trek up the mountain, they fear the unknown. It is difficult to move forward on an uncertain path that may well lead to a painful and uncertain future. Although family members, friends, and colleagues may fill up the space around us, the deep feeling of isolation remains.

The cancer experience produces mood swings. During the diagnostic phase we are deep in the blues. We see the mountain looming before us and wonder how we can even begin to confront it. Then we move into treatment and encounter fellow cancer patients and experience the unlikely communitas of the treatment room. During treatment we suddenly don't feel so alone. The anxieties we feel are a bit easier to bear. After a period of time, however, most cancer treatments come to an end. Our regimen of medicines and radiation has reduced the tumor. They may have even eliminated the cancer cells in our blood stream, bone marrow, or lymphatic system.

Even if we have achieved remission (more on this state later) and are symptom- and cancer-free, we know that our cancer may well return. As we leave the camaraderie of the treatment room, we ironically feel a sense of loss—a loss of communitas, one that often brings periods of depression.

In the world of cancer, the post-treatment blues are quite common. As the late Susan Sontag suggested, once we've spent time in the Kingdom of the Sick, we can't return completely to the Kingdom of the Healthy. That realization plunges most cancer patients into a state of sadness. But recognition and acceptance of this state are two steps to reclaiming a full life.

The transition from treatment to remission is a difficult one. Most cancer centers are sensitive to these transitional difficulties. Most of them employ skilled clinical social workers who can offer much-needed support. There is also a wealth of information on post-treatment depression. Here are a few to consider when someone is feeling the post-treatment blues.

RESOURCES ON POST-TREATMENT BLUES

1.   Mayo Clinic Staff. *Cancer survivors: Managing your emotions after cancer treatment.* www.mayoclinic.org/diseases-conditions/cancer/in-depth/...

2.   Cancer Survivors Network. 2010. *Post Cancer Depression.* http://csn.cancer.org/node/150731

3.   Jan Hoffman. 2013. *Anxiety Lingers Long After Cancer,* The New York Times, July 12, 2013. http://well.blogs.nytimes.com/2013/07/12/anxiety-lingers-long-after-cancer/

4.   American Cancer Society. 2014. *Anxiety, Fear, and Depression.* http://www.cancer.org/treatment/treatmentsandsideeffects/emotionalsideeffects/anxietyfearanddepression/anxiety-fear-and-depression-toc.

5.   Chen, Allen M. MD 2013, Depression up in post-radiation head and neck cancer survivors. Aug. 15 in *JAMA Otolaryngology-Head & Neck Surgery.*

6.   Dr. Frances Goodhart and Lucy Atkins. 2011 (June 14).

7.   Updated: 01:46 EST, 14 June 2011. *The downside of beating cancer.* http://www.dailymail.co.uk/health/article-2003214/Cancer-survivors-Depression-exhaustion-anger-downside-beating-disease.html#ixzz3M6IenJbZ .

8.   National Cancer Institute. *Depression (PDQ®).* http://www.cancer.gov/cancertopics/pdq/supportivecare/depression/HealthProfessional/page1/AllPages/Print.

9.   The Sunday Express 2010 (November 28) *Post-cancer depression: Darkness after dawn.* http://www.express.co.uk/life-style/health/214685/Post-cancer-depression-Darkness-after-dawn.

10.   LymphomaInfo.net. 2014. *Depression and Anxiety after Cancer Treatment.* http://www.lymphomainfo.net/videos/treatment/depression-and-anxiety-after-cancer-treatment.

11.   Kathy-Ellen Kups, 2007. Depression after cancer. *Everyday Health.* http://www.everydayhealth.com/columns/kathy-ellen-kups-life-with-breast-cancer/depression-after-cancer/

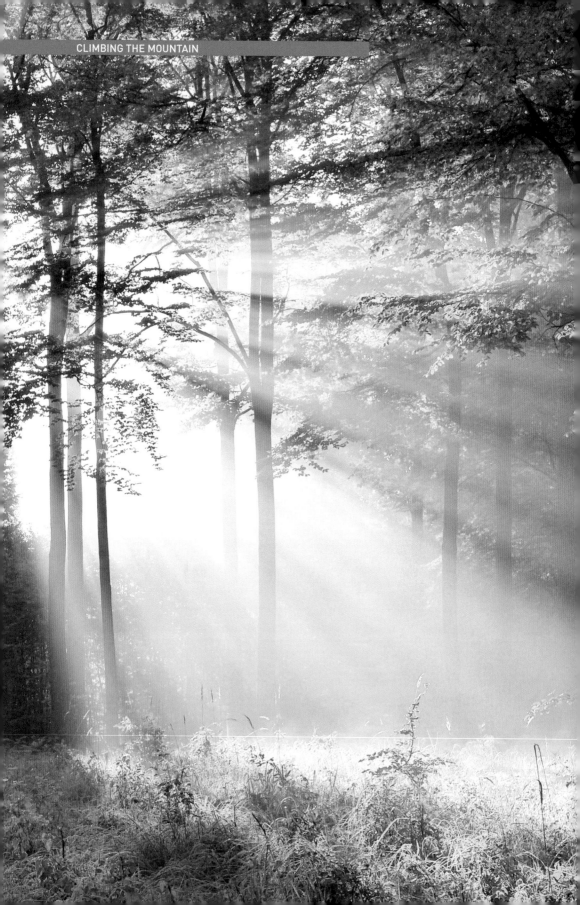

PART THREE:

Remission

PART THREE:

Remission

In this final part of the book, we consider the dynamics of remission, a subject that is under-represented in writing about the cancer experience. Most writers who reflect about cancer focus on the stresses and strains of diagnosis and treatment. Remission is a slippery slope. It is a space between health and illness, a place in which our prognosis is uncertain. In the chapters in this part of the book, we consider how best to confront these existential uncertainties. In Chapter 14, we describe the contours of remission's indeterminacy. In Chapter 15, we explore the creative possibilities that remission presents to us. In Chapter 16, we ponder the issue of well-being. What is it? Can it be measured? How can cancer patients experience it? The drama of oncological check-ups, which are periodic rituals, are explored in Chapter 17. In the Epilogue, we consider living fully and living well within our limitations.

14 THE POWER OF INDETERMINACY

Most people like stories that are clear, concrete, and well told. A good story tends to have a gripping beginning, an engaging plot full of memorable characters, and an end that presents a clear resolution—often a happy ending. In science, people prefer clear and resolute expression. A powerful argument has a concrete introduction, a presentation of results, a discussion of those results, and a concise conclusion—the scientific version of a happy ending.

The same can be said of our orientation to health and well-being. For most people, good health is a steady state; it is what we experience and expect of everyday life. When we develop symptoms of illness—aches, pains, and fevers—they compel us to visit a doctor, who prescribes treatment—a course of antibiotics, the use of an inhaler, decongestants, or antihistamines—which we follow for a period of time during which our symptoms fade away. In the end, we return to our state of health until we get sick again and go through the same routine again and

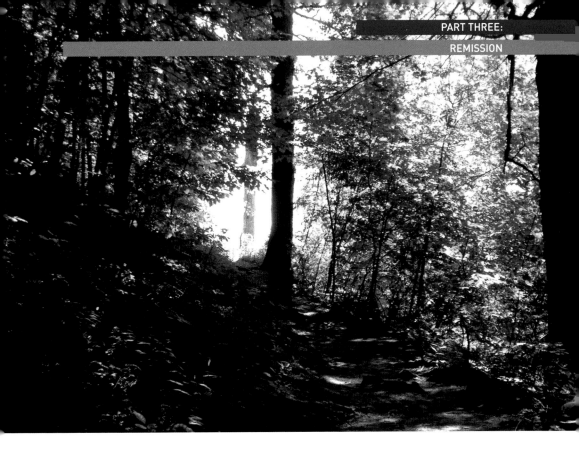

again. Most people live in the village of the healthy (see Stoller 2004). In the village people do not usually think about issues of health and well-being. We go to work, eat, celebrate, and take vacations. We certainly encounter problems on this path. There may be stress or conflicts at work. There may also be familial problems—concerns about our children, relatives and friends, and differences of opinion. Periodically we get sick, and then get better—until we develop a serious illness.

If we contract a chronic disease or disorder that has no cure, a condition that can be "managed" but not "eradicated," then everything changes. If we are diagnosed with most cancers, rheumatoid arthritis, most auto-immune disorders (like lupus and Guillaume Barr syndrome), or genetic disorders (like sickle cell anemia and Tay-Sachs disease), we enter a different village—the village of the sick. Treatments for these diseases cannot promise a return to the steady state of heath—only an alleviation of symptoms that are likely to return at some ill-defined point in the future. We call this remission. Millions of people live in what sociologist Arthur Frank calls "The Remission Society."

Remission makes climbing the mountain even more difficult. It is a slippery slope. Here's how Dr. Ed Zimney defines remission (in his blog, Dr. Ed's Medical Report):

Complete remission means that there are no symptoms and no signs that can be identified to indicate the presence of cancer. However, even when a person is in remission, there may be microscopic collections of cancer cells that cannot be identified by current techniques. This means that even if a person is in remission, they may, at some future time, experience a recurrence of their cancer.

Partial remission means that a large percentage of the signs and symptoms of cancer are gone, but some still remain. Complete remission would therefore be better than partial remission because with partial remission the chances of recurrence are higher. (http://www.everydayhealth.com/columns/zimney-health-and-medical-news-you-can-use/cancer-cure-vs-remission/)

In a more concrete fashion, the term remission:

...comes from the verb to remit, which can refer to, among other things, states of relief, abatement, hiatus, interruption, respite, stoppage and subsidence. Except for stoppage, none of the states connoted by remission signifies a condition of permanence. Such words as *relief, abatement, interruption, respite* and *subsidence* suggest an eventual return to a preexisting state. *Hiatus* refers to a temporary place between what was and what will be. Even stoppage betrays an indirect impermanence. In the end remission means spending years 'being on hold,' 'waiting for the other shoe to drop,' or 'sitting on your hands.' It is not an easy place to be. (Stoller 2004: 1818-82)

In other words, remission puts us in a place between health and disease—an indeterminate space that defies our conventional routines.

The texture of remission is beautifully captured in a chapter of Claude Levi-Strauss's famous anthropological memoir, *Tristes Tropiques*, the chronicle of his early research trip to Brazil in the 1930s. On his way from France to Brazil, Levi-

Strauss's ship passes through an intertropical zone known as the doldrums. It is a dead zone where the wind stops—a space that is between the Old and New Worlds. When sailors traversed the doldrums in tall ships, they knew that once they entered the zone, it would be difficult to turn around and go back to their world. Once in the doldrums, they would have to drift for indeterminate periods of time. They would remain physically and existentially between the worlds until they picked up the southern trade winds that would carry them to their destination from which they might return, forever changed by their confrontation with the New World.

This drifting in a space between the old and the new is not unlike the state of remission. During remission, we pass beyond what we know and drift into a space that has no distinct boundaries and no concrete destination. Once in remission, we enter the "village of the sick." In this village of the sick, everyone shares one characteristic: we are in remission from a disease that has no cure. We look back to our old lives in the village of the healthy and realize that we can never fully return to that place. Our time in the village of sick has changed us; it has put us in an indeterminate state that, unlike a good story, has no clear-cut beginnings or endings. Our fellow patients usually understand this life of living betwixt and between. As we mentioned in Chapter 7, the anthropologist Victor Turner suggested everyone is subject to living betwixt and between. Whenever we participate in a rite of passage, such as a birth, a confirmation, a graduation, a marriage, or a divorce, we enter a state in which we are between two recognized identities. Before a wedding, for example, we are single. During the ceremony, we are somewhere between being single and married. After the ceremony, we are married—a new identity. Turner called this state "liminality." In his view, liminality is a temporary state. We are betwixt and between during the performance of a ritual. Once that ceremony is complete, we return to a more or less "normal" state. When we are in remission, however, we enter the difficult state of "continuous liminality," in which the complexities of being everywhere and nowhere continue indefinitely.

Immigrants often find themselves in a state of continuous liminality. They have left their natal countries and never quite feel at "home" in the country to which they immigrated. Even if they return to the country of their birth, their time "away" will change their sense of their home country. To quote the title of a famous Thomas Wolfe novel: *You Can't Go Home Again.*

People who are in remission often find themselves in a similar state. We want to return to the village of the healthy. We want to resume our old lives. But we cannot. We may leave the village of the sick and even enter the village of the healthy to visit. Even though such a visit is heartwarming, we cannot feel fully at home. Our loved ones often don't fully understand our experience in the village of the sick.

JOHN'S STATE OF REMISSION

As we mentioned in chapter 13, John, like many cancer patients, experienced a bout of post-treatment depression. When his oncologist told him that he was in remission, he felt temporary elation. He was going to live free of cancer symptoms and the devastating effects of chemotherapy. That alone was cause for celebration. John's law firm arranged a remission party. He and Beth celebrated privately with a bottle of champagne. Once the initial relief and festivities were over, John began to feel a nagging anxiety. He thought long and hard about his life. He re-evaluated how he had spent his days. Some of his past activities no longer interested him. At work, he no longer felt that burning sense of competitiveness. The desire to "get ahead" had dissipated. He no longer saw any reason to continue to work long, grueling hours. He even thought of leaving his law firm, or perhaps working part-time. He thought about devoting some of his time to working as a pro bono poverty lawyer—one of his youthful dreams that had been swept aside. He also wanted to continue practicing yoga and meditation. He wanted to hike and bike in nature—activities that brought him peace and pleasure.

As he moved deeper into remission, John tried not to dwell on the uncertainty of his life. After all, all life was uncertain. He began to read about remission. He read about the Sufi mystic al-Arabia, a medieval thinker who wondered about the space between things—the spaces that we encounter in remission. Al-Arabia said that the indeterminate spaces between things make us nervous and unsure of ourselves. In that space that is everywhere and nowhere, we confront the power of the imagination—the power to contour a new life, the creativity to be in the moment. John found these ideas appealing.

His reading, yoga, and meditation made him more appreciative of the present—the here and now. He felt grateful for his state of remission—a pain-free space—and would try to take advantage of the physical and emotional energy that now surged through his being.

BOOKS ON CANCER AND REMISSION

There are hundreds of books about the experience of cancer remission. Many promise quick fixes to cure cancer and suggest that such-and-such a diet may prevent the recurrence of cancer. The books we list below, however, are a small sample of texts that consider both the philosophical and medical dimensions of remission.

1. Frank, Arthur W. 1995. *The Wounded Storyteller.* University of Chicago Press.
2. Turner, Kelly. 2014. Radical Remission. New York: HarperOne.
3. Williams, Pat, and Pat Denney 2014. *The Mission is Remission.* HCI Books.
4. Stoller, Paul 2004. *Stranger in the Village of the Sick.* Boston: Beacon Books
5. Stoller, Paul 2014. *Yaya's Story: The Quest for Well-Being in the World.* Chicago: The University of Chicago Press.
6. Mukherjee, Sidartha. 2010. *The Emperor of All Maladies.* New York: Scribner.
7. Servan-Schreiber, David. 2008. *Anti-Cancer: A New Way of Life.* New York: Viking.
8. Remen, Rachel Naomi. 2001. *My Grandfather's Blessings: Stories of Strength, Refuge and Belonging.* New York: Penguin.

15 EXERCISING CREATIVITY

When we climb the mountain, we each experience unique challenges. There are always conventional paths available that others have travelled, paths free of rocks and branches. Some of these paths may be easy; others more difficult. Some paths may offer beautiful views, others more unconventional outlooks. The unconventional ones are often less trodden and more challenging; at the same time they are also more likely to provide rich rewards.

In the world of cancer, there are many paths up the mountain. Some people choose conventional routes of treatment; others combine the conventional with the innovative. There are cancer patients who even select radical approaches to cancer treatment. When we enter remission, the world becomes less clear-cut. When we enter remission and are free of symptoms and side effects, we once again face a new path up the mountain. Remission offers an expansion of possibilities—new ways to continue on life's path.

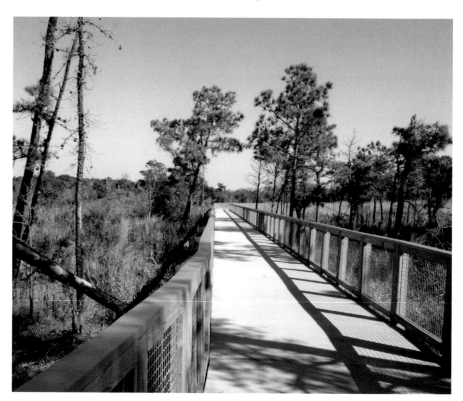

Sometimes the proliferation of choices can be overwhelming. In remission we are given a new lease on life, if only for an indeterminate amount of time. It's like being given a chance to refashion life and begin anew. What an opportunity! What a burden! We may become panicked with the fear that we might waste this new opportunity.

For many people the challenge of a new life is too stressful. In these cases, cancer patients return to their old habits and patterns. But even this choice is difficult because the experience of cancer changes everything. Most people in remission resume their lives but with an altered set of priorities. A hard-driving business executive may take a softer approach to management. A scholar may shift his or her priorities from cutting-edge research to teaching effectively. A writer may shift his or her expository emphasis from complex analysis or intricate plots to simple storytelling. And then there are people who want to make a radical break from a previous life. They may decide to live or work in a bungalow on an exotic beach or next to a bucolic lake. They may relocate to a bustling city. In some cases remission is a trigger for early (or not so early) retirement, which could mean travel and adventure.

Regardless of the path, remission is a space between things, an indeterminate arena of fuzzy beginnings and uncertain ends. It can also be a time of creativity and self-expansion. Here's what the medieval Andalusian Sufi mystic, Al-Arabi, says about the spaces between things (remission spaces). For him the between is

> Something that separates…two things, while never going to one side…as, for example, the line that separates shadow from sun light. God says, 'he let forth the two seas that meet together, between a barzakh (bridge) they do not overpass (Koran 55:19); in other words one sea does not mix with the other…Any two adjacent things are in need of barzakh, which is neither one nor the other but which possesses the power…of both. The barzakh is something that separates a known from an unknown, an existent from a non-existent, a negated from an affirmed, an intelligible from a non-intelligible (Crapanzano 2003, 57-58; see also Chittick 1989)

As we have said, dwelling between things can be off-putting and downright frightening, such as when a cancer patient has completed treatment and is attempting to confront the ambiguous space between health and illness. And yet, if we exercise our imagination, the unsettling spaces between things can become arenas of creative discovery. In the words of anthropologist Vincent Crapanzano (2003:58) the between (or the liminal)

> ...has often been likened to a dream. It suggests imaginative possibilities that are not necessarily available to us in everyday life. Through paradox, ambiguity, contradiction, bizarre, exaggerated, and at times grotesque symbols, masks, and figurines, and the evocation of transcendent realities, mystery and supernatural powers, the liminal offers us a view of the world to which we are normally blinded by the usual structures of social and cultural life.

The between, then, "can be a space of creative imagination, of provocative linkages, of *barzakh*, and of personal empowerment" (Stoller 2008:6). It can be a creative space for writers, scholars, and filmmakers as well as for cancer patients entering remission. The emotional key here is our willingness to take the existential risk of exercising our creativity.

In "Cancer Survivors Discover Personal Growth," Kathryn Johnson, Ph.D. wrote:

> Cancer changes you. That's an understatement, isn't it? Along with physical changes—like surgical scars or lingering after-effects—there are emotional and spiritual changes. The journey of a person with cancer is often compared to the archetypal "hero's journey," where the main character in a story overcomes huge challenges to attain life-changing gifts. It's in those life-changing gifts—those emotional and spiritual changes—where cancer survivors often find new possibilities and new meaning in life. We call it "post-traumatic growth."

COMMON AREAS OF POST-TRAUMATIC GROWTH

Obviously, few of us would choose a traumatic event as an avenue for growth. But, when faced with the struggle to make sense of a cancer diagnosis, people are forced to question their fundamental assumptions about the world. And, often, they do discover new life-changing gifts of personal growth, including:

New possibilities for life. Cancer survivors often set new goals and priorities. They feel more strongly about believing and investing in themselves and others. They have a new commitment to their physical health. They work on checking things off their bucket list. They understand they can't assume the future they planned on will be there.

Relating to others. Surviving cancer gives a whole new meaning to "don't sweat the small stuff." Many cancer survivors no longer get bogged down in petty personal squabbles. Rather, they choose to focus on improving personal relationships and having greater empathy for others.

Recognizing personal strengths. Traumatic experiences really can make a person stronger. Cancer survivors prove again and again that personal growth, resilience and the power to overcome difficult circumstances are possible and probable. Sometimes, surviving cancer makes a person recognize they have the strength to leave a stressful job or a bad relationship to chart a new and more fulfilling course.

Greater appreciation for life. Facing cancer means facing one's own mortality. Surviving cancer provides a new perspective and greater appreciation for life. Someone who previously contemplated suicide might now value and celebrate the gift of life every second of every day. (http://www.provcancerblog.org/2013/10/cancer-survivors-discover-personal-growth/)

JOHN CONFRONTS A SET OF NEW POSSIBILITIES

John's diagnosis and treatment path compelled him open his mind to a variety of options that we have discussed in this book: yoga, meditation, massage, and reflexology. Each of these expanded the view of his life. He now decided that he could combat his "blue" days by learning French—something he had always wanted to do. He had already decided to keep practicing law and continue his hobbies, but he wanted to do more with this new life betwixt and between health and illness.

As a teenager, John had always wanted to learn French and spend time in Paris. But life intervened. Cancer made John realize that it was now or never. He talked with Beth about how to begin his new project. They decided to plan a trip to Europe. This trip would give John a strong incentive to learn French.

John signed up for an introductory adult education French class at his local college. The class met one night a week. Surprisingly, he very much enjoyed the class, which consisted of a diverse group people of all ages and backgrounds.

Outside of class, John listened to French lessons while on the treadmill at the gym. He also watched the news on the local French language station.

One of John's classmates was Jane, a 72-year-old who had always dreamed of traveling to Paris. Like John, she also scheduled a trip to France. Also like John, she wanted to learn as much French as possible before setting foot in the City of Light.

"I can't wait to read a menu and order my dinner in Paris."

John greatly enjoyed his new pursuit. He also began to study and occasionally cook French food. Every two weeks, he and Beth would watch a French film with subtitles. John got excited when he began to understand some of the dialogue.

THE BENEFITS OF CREATIVITY AND PERSONAL GROWTH

The creativity process generates new ideas and triggers new possibilities. Creativity is inventive, novel, and original, but it has a unique meaning for each person. There are many paths to the wonders of creativity. However you might define them, creative activities can enrich your life.

For many other cancer patients, remission can be a time in life that promotes the opportunity to try something new: study a foreign language, write a short story, learn how to draw or how to throw a pot, take up weaving or knitting, travel to an exotic location, or enroll in a cooking class. It is a time when the senses are heightened, when the meaning of life is contemplated, and when former dreams are revisited. It can be a time to explore the passions that we never had a chance to pursue. Some creative strategies include:

1. **Do what you are under-skilled to do** – if you know pretty well what you are doing you are probably jaded by now.
2. **Do not be defensive about your ideas** – that's when you think your ideas are too silly and defy common sense.
3. **Imagine, visualize, and persevere**
4. **Allow randomness**
5. **Bring new life to old ideas** – there are no new ideas, really. But there are new combinations of old ideas.
6. **Face your fears** and anxieties
7. **Be wrong**
8. **Collaborate** – there is someone out there in the world right now who is thinking about the same things you are. Why not put your brains together?
9. **Stretch ideas** – stretching your mind and ideas means pushing them to go where they don't want to go. It hurts like doing the splits. But it opens you up to new possibilities.
10. **Listen to yourself**

http://fundersandfounders.com/how-to-be-creative-31-ways/

We list below several resources on the human imagination and creative impulse.

1. Chittick, W.C. 1989. *The Sufi Path of Knowledge.* State University of New York Press.
2. Crapanzano, Vincent 2003. *Imaginative Horizons.* University of Chicago Press.

3. Csikszentmihalyi, Mihaly. 1997. *Creativity: Flow and the Psychology of Discovery and Invention*. New York: Harper Perennial.

4. Loori, John Daido. 2005. *The Zen of Creativity: Cultivating Your Artistic Life*. New York: Ballatine Books.

5. Csikszentmihalyi, Mihaly 2013, *Creativity: The Psychology of Discovery and Invention*. New York: Harper Perennial.

6. Moreno Pl and AL Stanton 2013. Personal growth during the experience of advanced cancer: a systematic review. *Cancer J*. 2013 Sep-Oct;19(5):421-30. doi: 10.1097/PPO.ob013e3182a5bbe7.

7. Phillips, Jan, 2005. *The Art of Original Thinking: The Making of a Thought Leader*. (9th Element Press)

8. Wilson, Anthony. 2013. *Remission Anniversary Seven*. http://anthonywilsonpoetry.com/category/remission/page/3/

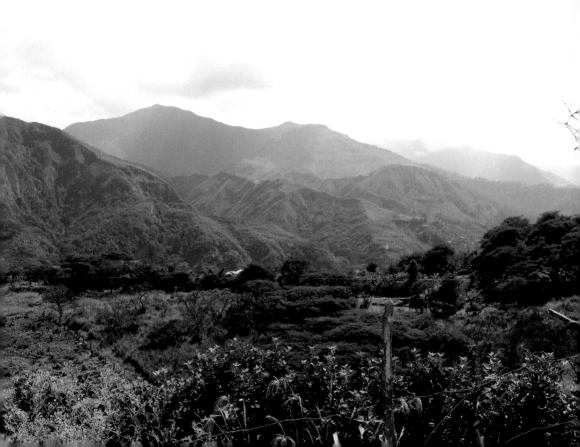

16 WELL-BEING ALONG THE PATH

In many respects, John's story epitomizes a positive response to cancer. He read widely about cancer so that he could manage his treatment as much as possible. He was lucky. He did so with the considerable emotional and social support of his wife and friends. It's hard to make life and death decisions in a social vacuum. Because they informed themselves, John and Beth could insightfully discuss John's physical and emotional concerns about diagnosis and treatment.

Although a cancer diagnosis turned John's world upside down, he and Beth tried to cope with a stressful and difficult situation with as much normalcy as possible. John tried to understand what was happening to him. He tried to stay informed and understand his treatment options. He experimented with new treatment interventions that could help him cope with the potentially devastating negative side effects of cancer treatment. As we have documented, he explored a variety of complementary measures and strategies to reduce the impact of chemotherapy and immunotherapy. He continued to exercise as much as he could at his local gym. Even if he felt tired, he dragged himself to the trail near his house so that he could connect with nature. Walking in the forest and hearing the sound of the wind rustling through the leaves brought him peace.

As we have stated, John was able to continue his work at the law firm, eventually on a part-time basis. Throughout his treatment, John struggled not to let his illness control his life. For many patients, it is exceedingly difficult to maintain their autonomy. Like most patients, John did not want to surrender himself completely to his illness. Following the advice of Beth and others, John tried meditation, yoga, and massage and reflexology during the treatment period. He attended a support group. These activities did indeed help him. They made him feel less isolated and less alone on the path up the mountain.

When John entered remission, he, like many cancer patients, felt let-down. He also felt a creeping anxiety and even depression. He had achieved his goal, but he also missed the camaraderie of the treatment room. He longed to spend more time with people who understood his pain and anxiety. Remission was new territory; it offered a new path.

After conversations with Beth and his friends, John decided to continue with what had worked during treatment. He maintained his complementary treatments. He continued to try to stay active. He went back to work full-time. John gradually noticed that he was more fully engaged in life. His orientation to work had changed. As a senior member of the firm, he found that he now enjoyed spending more time with the younger associates. Mentoring became more important to him. He wanted to instill in them a respect for the law, something that had taken him a long time to learn. He also wanted to devote some of his time to pro bono work to help make a contribution to his community.

Remission also made John conscious of life's limits. He knew that his cancer could return at any time, which meant that he didn't want whatever time he had left to be wasted. He also wanted to make his life as creative and meaningful as possible. He felt very philosophical about his new outlook. "It's like walking up a mountain," he told Beth. "The higher up we go, the greater our awareness of what's important in life. When you reach the top, maybe that's when all of the paths converge and things make sense. Maybe then we feel a sense of comfort."

THE PATHS OF REMISSION

As John's cancer experience suggests, remission brings the texture of life into sharp relief. From this vantage point, life is a series of paths, all of which end in forks in the road. At each fork on the path, everyone must decide which new path to take. Do we move left on a path that leads to a mountain, or do we turn right on a path that leads to a forest? Our choices shape the direction of our future. The fork in the road is a space filled with uncertainty, for it is here that we choose our fate. It is a point of anxiety and reflection that all of us must negotiate on life's path.

Some people call the fork in the road a point of misfortune. Given the considerable challenges of walking a path that may be filled with poverty, illness, disappointment, and misfortune, how can we cope with the challenges of life and not become depressed?

Here's one way of coping with the stresses of serious illness and the uncertainties of remission:

> Taking into consideration individual differences in how people react to sickness, Songhay culture [in the Republic of Niger] promotes a much less individualistic approach to illness and death. Finding themselves in the shadows cast by the natural forces of life and death, the Songhay are taught to think that they are relatively insignificant beings—trickles...in the stream of history. Swept up in the strong current of life, many Songhay think that life is like a loan that can never be fully repaid. On the given due date, you must make a payment, but you can never pay off the principal. You hope that your payments make a lasting contribution to your friends, family, and community. This kind of cultural orientation breeds considerable respect for the forces of the universe, including the ongoing presence of illness in the body. If a Songhay develops a serious illness like cancer, he or she is likely to build respect for it. Respect for cancer—or any illness—does not mean that you meekly submit to the ravages of disease....illness is accepted as an ongoing part of life. When illness appears, it presents one with limitations, but if it is possible to accept the limitations and work within their parameters, one can...create a degree of comfort in uncomfortable circumstances (Stoller 2004: 191).

Put another way, we may face many life-limiting obstacles in our lives, but those difficulties need not prevent us from feeling degrees of comfort—even during chemotherapy sessions or during the silently uncertain hours that unfold during remission—in uncomfortable situations. For many of us, an acknowledgment of our limitations is an acknowledgment of weakness. Such an orientation can make confronting an illness with no cure—or mortality itself—even more unbearable. Even so, the capacity to respect illness (and its set of physical and emotional limitations) is an important element in the pursuit of well-being, an ever-elusive aspect of human experience.

Feelings of well-being are often fleeting and can emerge in any situation. Humanistic psychologists have introduced the notion of "peak experiences," moments when we experience feelings of complete well-being. For cancer patients facing mortality, such moments can emerge when they come to peaceful terms with the past and present. Moments of well-being can be experienced in childhood when we are fully engaged in play or in adulthood during a walk on a sunny afternoon. They can also be experienced during cancer treatments or even when facing the end of our lives. The key is to fully savor these moments. Studies have shown that people report feelings of well-being and happiness even when they are struggling with a chronic illness like cancer.

As John's case illustrates, cancer remission brings both relief and anxiety. Treatment is over, at least for now, but for how long? You still have regular, stress-producing check-ups. Even so, many cancer patients like John also realize that life is to be lived as fully as possible. Below are some tips for coping with remission:

+ Accept your anxiety and fear and realize that everyone experiences them
+ Share your fears
+ Stay informed
+ Live a healthy lifestyle
+ Exercise
+ Eat a good diet
+ Drink moderately
+ Manage your stress
+ Spend time with those who love you
+ Enjoy your hobbies, work, and activities
+ Use humor as a coping mechanism
+ Ask for help

http://www.cancer.net/survivorship/life-after-cancer/coping-fear-recurrence

RESOURCES ON CANCER AND WELL-BEING

1. Barr, Nikki. 2014. Cancer and Bringing Peace Back In: *Patients, Survivors, Caregivers*. http://canceremotionalwellbeing. com/2014/03/cancer-and-bringing-peace-back-in-patients-survivors-caregivers/;
2. O'Donnell, Lucy. 2014. *Emotional Well-being and Cancer*. www. psychologytoday.com/blog/cancer-is-teacher/201411/emotional-well-being-and-cancer)
3. Office of Cancer Survivorship, National Institute of Health. 2014. *Health and Well-Being After Cancer* http://cancercontrol.cancer. govthe /ocs/resources/health-after-cancer.html;
4. Stoller, Paul. 2014. *Yaya's Story: The Quest for Well-Being in the World*. Chicago: The University of Chicago Press.
5. Stoller, Paul. 2015. *Well-being in the World*. The Huffington Post, February 5 edition.

17 REMISSION RITES

The end of John's treatment was approaching. After a grueling nine-month program of chemotherapy and immunotherapy, John's oncologist told him that there was no discernible trace of cancer in his body. The news made John and his family very happy. He celebrated with a bottle of champagne!

For a few weeks, John floated through his days. He felt light, happy, and renewed. He refocused his energies on his job, tried to be extra helpful around the house, cleaned out his study, and walked slowly, smelling the roses. Gradually, however, he came to the realization that remission is also a scary time, and it is a slippery slope for cancer patients. Many of John's family, friends, loved ones, and colleagues thought that remission meant that he was cured of cancer, which, of course, is not the case for most cancers. As stated previously, remission places people in the indeterminate space between health and illness—a space that can be fraught with doubt, anxiety, and fear. Patients like John live in an in-between state, because they are no longer officially "ill," and they are no longer on a path to regain their "health," but at the same time they are also cancer "survivors,"with all of the accompanying identity issues and behaviors that go along with this in-between place.

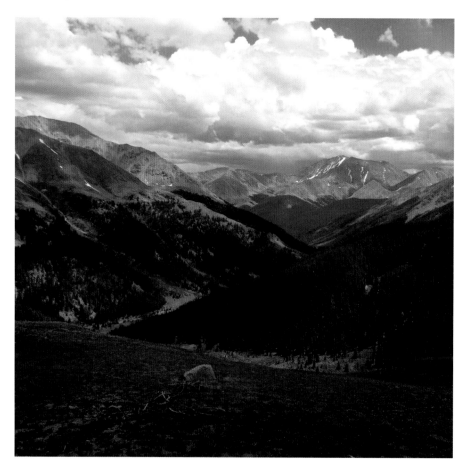

REMISSION TIMELINES

Remission is a state during which diseases are "managed." During this period of physical and emotional limbo, cancer patients go for checkups at arranged intervals. Checkups, tests, and doctor's visits constitute remission rites. In most cases, these rites include blood work, a physical examination, and perhaps a CT scan. These are procedures that produce medical evidence that is evaluated and discussed during a visit to a physician. If the results of these rites are "good," we remain in remission, which means that will go through a similar set of remission rites three months, six months, or one year later. If the results of the checkup are not "good," we reenter treatment, hoping again, like Sisyphus, for a return to the state of remission.

Despite the opportunities that it can afford, remission is nonetheless sobering and taxing. However, as cancer patients move along, the time between remission rites can become more or less normal. Everyday life can take on a pleasant routine. Friends and family members no longer have to think so much about their loved one's disease.

Some people consider those who have "beaten" cancer as "survivors." Given this kind of patient narrative, cancer patients sometimes fall into the false consciousness of having toughed it out, of having survived a painful ordeal, of having fought the enemy and won.

JOHN'S REMISSION RITES

John sometimes included himself in that all-too-common "survivor" category. Remission gave him a new confidence. As previous chapters have indicated, John's illness had also resulted in personal growth and development. He now practiced yoga and meditation. He studied French. He and Beth travelled more than they had before John's diagnosis and treatment. He was more relaxed and supportive of others in his work. He was very grateful for these changes in his life. The changes exacted a cost, however. John knew that he would have to live with the uncertainties that cancer had brought into his life. Would it return?

When his five-year cancer-free anniversary arrived, John felt gratitude for an unexpected extension of his life. His zest for whatever time he had left continued. By then he knew that the uncertainties of remission would slow him down but not stop him. Even so, when the dates for his remission rites approached, every six months, John felt anxious and stressed. The remission rite is not unlike a

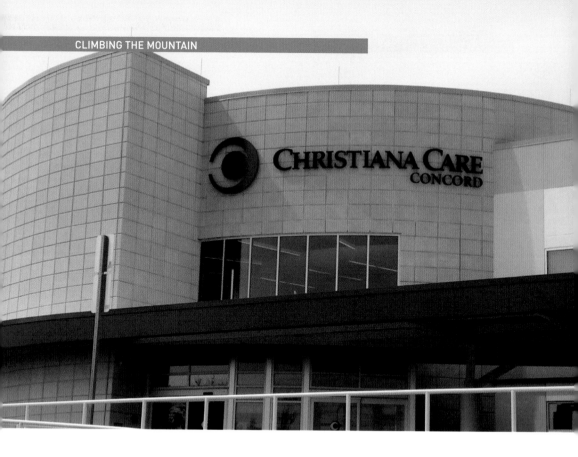

trial—the verdict of which can unalterably change our lives. Even though John had become a five-year remission-rite veteran, the prospect of going once again to The Cancer Center frightened him.

His oncologist, who had become a friend, chatted about their mutual interest in travelling, their families and friends, and other interests. On these visits John's doctor asked routine questions about night sweats and unusual lumps, none of which he had experienced. During the visit five years after John's initial diagnosis, the doctor palpated John's body, looking for swollen lymph nodes or other potential abnormalities—never a pleasant experience, especially if the physician finds something unexpected and says:

"Let me feel that again." He examined John's underarms and elbow a second time. "You've got some swollen nodes. They're tiny, but they're there."

This exchange was almost identical to the one John had had five years earlier when his primary care physician discovered an abdominal tumor. John remembered all too well how his life had been turned upside down in a matter of seconds. These swollen nodes might have resulted from an infection or from the scratches John would routinely get from walking along the trails near his house. But at the same time, the swollen nodes might be a signal of cancer's return.

John's oncologist suggested that they wait to see if the nodes persisted. Trying his best to live with such uncertainty, which is difficult, John returned to The Cancer Center one month later. Physical examination revealed the ongoing presence of the nodes. John's oncologist insisted on ordering blood work and a CT scan, which, due to scheduling issues, had to be delayed. John's life had yet again taken an unexpected and unwanted twist, reminding him once again of remission's innumerable difficulties. John tried to carry on. He succeeded to some extent, but he couldn't completely shake the dread of cancer's potential return.

John worried about the new scan. What would the results reveal? Would he again be a regular guest in the treatment room? As it turned out, the CT scan was normal, which was great news—definitely worth more champagne. But John had become a realist. He knew that remission rites would be a permanent feature of his future, which meant that his existential limbo would persist.

COPING WITH REMISSION

Remission is indeterminate. If a person has a cancer without a cure, chances are that it will return. Even so, we can learn to live—and live well—in remission. Beyond its stresses and strains, remission, as we have suggested, can be a space of great creativity and insight, an arena of what the poet John Keats called "negative capability"—learning to live with psychological and physical uncertainties.

In a letter to his brother, Keats wrote:

> At once it struck me, what quality went to form a Man of Achievement, especially in literature, and which Shakespeare possessed so enormously—I mean Negative Capability, that is when man is capable of being in uncertainties. Mysteries, doubts, without any irritable reaching after fact and reason. [http://www.keatsian.co.uk/negative-capability.php]

Being a remission-rite adept, however, did not make John—or anyone else—a "fighter," a "warrior," or a "survivor." Like most cancer patients, the realities of remission make cancer patients individuals who are simply trying to live fully within the limits of their circumstances.

There is a large literature consisting of both scientific studies and self-help guides that provide information on coping with remission—for cancer patients and their families. There is no one correct way of coping with remission, any more than there is one way of treating cancer. Suggestions for coping with remission are similar to other suggestions we have made for coping with diagnosis and treatment.

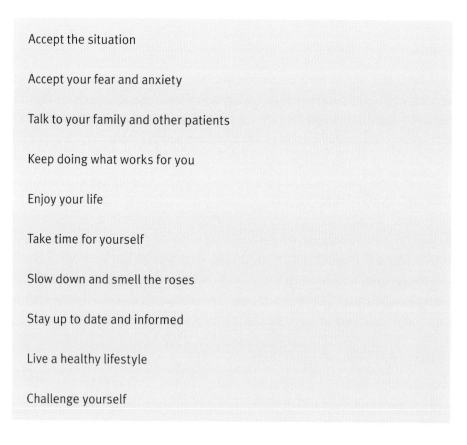

Accept the situation

Accept your fear and anxiety

Talk to your family and other patients

Keep doing what works for you

Enjoy your life

Take time for yourself

Slow down and smell the roses

Stay up to date and informed

Live a healthy lifestyle

Challenge yourself

COPING RESOURCES

1. Buchsel, P.C. (2009). "Survivorship issues in hematopoietic stem cell transplantation. Seminars in Oncology Nursing., 25(2) 159-169.

2. Cancer. Net. 2015. Coping With Fear of Recurrence. http://www.cancer.net/survivorship/life-after-cancer/coping-fear-recurrence

3. Castellino, S., Melissa & Hudson, M. "Health issues in survivors of childhood cancer." Southern Medical Journal 95 (2002): 977-984.

4. Children's Oncology Group Long-Term Follow-Up Guidelines for Survivors of Childhood, Adolescent, and Young Adult Cancers, Version 2.0 (including "Health Link: Reducing the Risk of Second Cancers") http://www.survivorshipguidelines.org/

5. Deeg, H. J., Schwartz, J L. Friedman, D., & Lessening, W. "Secondary malignancies after hemopoietic stem cell transplantation." Perspectives in Medical Science (September 29, 2003).

6. Hieb BA, Ogle SK, Meadows AT. "Second malignancies following treatment for childhood cancer." Survivors of Childhood and Adolescent Cancer 2nd edition Eds. C.L. Schwartz, W.L. Hobbie, L.S. Constine, K.S. Ruccione. Berlin: Springer, 2005, pp. 283-294.

7. Hudson, M. M., Merten, A. C., Yasui, Y, Hobbie, W., Chen, H. Gurney, et al. "Health status of adult long-term survivors of childhood cancer: A report from the childhood cancer survivor study." Journal of American Medical Association 290 12 (2003): 1583-1592.

8. LiveStrong Foundation 2015. Fear of Recurrence. http://www.livestrong.org/we-can-help/healthy-living-after-treatment/second-cancers/

9. Mayo Clinic 2015. When cancer returns: How to cope with cancer recurrence. http://www.mayoclinic.org/diseases-conditions/cancer/in-depth/cancer/ART-20044575

10. Morrison, C. H., "Early detection of cancer." Core Curriculum of Oncology Nursing. Eds. J. K. Itano & K. N. Talka. Philadelphia: W. B. Saunders Company, 2005. pp. 861-874.

11. Schulthies, Erin 2014. Making the Most of Depression Remission. http://www.healthyplace.com/blogs/

copingwithdepression/2014/04/making-the-most-of-depression-remission/.

12. "Secondary cancers: Incidence, risk factors, and management." Cancer.org. S. R. Rheingold, A. Neugut & N. T. Meadows. 29 September 2003 http://www.cancer.org

13. Wallace ML, Dombrovski AY, Morse JQ, Houck PR, Frank E, Alexopoulos GS, Reynolds CF 3rd, Schulz R. 2012. Coping with health stresses and remission from late-life depression in primary care: a two-year prospective study. Int J Geriatr Psychiatry. Feb 27(2):178-86. doi: 10.1002/gps.2706. Epub 2011 Ma

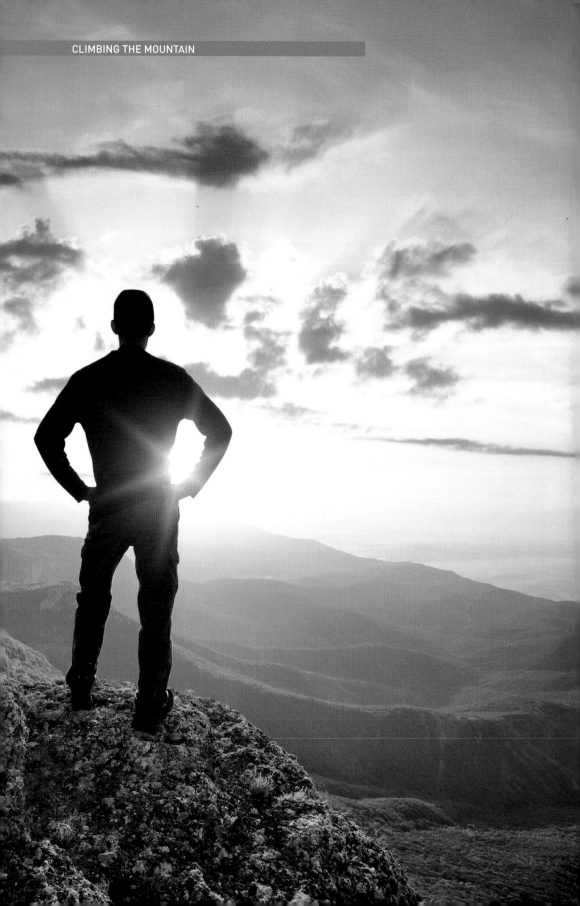

EPILOGUE:

Living Well in the World

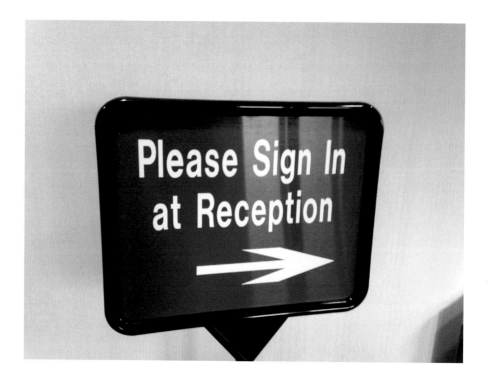

This book has focused on the story of one man who, in midlife, was confronted with a life-threatening chronic illness. We have attempted to document his struggle on the new and unexpected life path cancer forced him to follow. There are many possible life paths for each person, regardless of the state of his or her health and well-being. We have presented a few strategies that appear to help cancer patients along their path. Our list of suggestions is by no means complete or the right way for everyone. Each person must choose what works for him or her. In the end, the most important question we face is: How can we live well in the world? How can we live well regardless of what is happening to us? A significant part of our well-being is, after all, internal.

The question of living well in the world has long been at forefront of philosophical reflection. There is, of course, no clear answer to the question. The question of how to live well in the world is a cultural one. A person who grew up in Indonesia would have one path toward living well in the world. Someone in New York City or Berlin would have another distinct set of ideas about how to live well in the world. One element is beyond question: no matter our station in life or where we live, no matter our physical or mental state, everyone engages in the quest for well-being.

It has become clear that states of well-being and happiness do not necessarily depend on economic factors. It is also clear that it is difficult to measure indices of well-being. In the past ten years, psychologists have conducted surveys and developed exercises in "positive psychology." These attempt to focus on issues of happiness and well-being (see Seligman 2003). What are the factors, these researchers ask, that make life satisfying, enjoyable, and worth living?

Scholars have also developed objective indices to rank well-being. United Nations Human Development Index researchers use a matrix of objective well-being measurements, like per-capita income and life expectancy, to rate the "livability" of nations. These ratings, however, appear to have limited applicability. A December 19, 2012 Gallup survey, for example, found that:

The world's happiest people aren't in Qatar, the richest country by most measures. They aren't in Japan, the nation with the highest life expectancy. Canada, with its chart-topping percentage of college graduates, doesn't make the top 10.

A poll released Wednesday of nearly 150,000 people around the world says seven of the world's 10 countries with the most upbeat attitudes are in Latin America...

Many of the seven do poorly in traditional measures of well-being, like Guatemala, a country torn by decades of civil war followed by waves of gang-driven criminality that give it one of the highest homicide rates in the world. Guatemala sits just above Iraq on the United Nations' Human Development Index, a composite of life expectancy, education and per capita income. But it ranks seventh in positive emotions...

Prosperous nations can be deeply unhappy ones. And poverty-stricken ones are often awash in positivity, or at least a close approximation of it. (Weissenstein 2012)

This finding suggests that human well-being is captured less by objective economic or sociological indicators than by the quality of social relations—the texture of social life as it is lived.

LIVING WELL WITH SERIOUS ILLNESS

Serious illness, of course, presents a profound challenge to our struggle to live well in the world. As we have stated, illness is often accompanied by anxiety and depression, physical pain and discomfort, and emotional struggles. Cancer patients worry about side effects, missed or incomplete diagnoses, and poor treatment choices—not to mention the slow march toward a potentially painful and unpleasant death. There is nothing anyone can say to alleviate these thoughts and fears.

As we have suggested, however, a diagnosis of cancer is not a death sentence. In this book we have suggested how cancer patients can cope with their illness. Although many cancers have no cures, medical advancements have improved the situation considerably. Most cancers can be managed with an array of medical and technological interventions. People with cancer often find themselves in the "remission society" for longer and longer periods of time. As we have stated throughout this book, the state of remission is a difficult one. It is a space filled with happiness and gratitude, but also confusion and anxiety. Although most cancer patients are grateful to be in a state free of symptoms, they are still very much in the nebulous area between health and illness, a state in which cancer can return without warning.

We have suggested how cancer patients might cope with the challenges of diagnosis, treatment, and remission. We have put forward a number of ideas about how cancer patients might manage the considerable stress of diagnosis— of knowing that something is terribly wrong, but not knowing what that might be. We have stated that patients undergoing various treatments for cancer— chemotherapies, immunotherapies, and radiation—can take concrete measures to reduce the pain of harmful physical side effects and lessen the sting of debilitating depression. These concrete measures—regular exercise, communing with nature, yoga, meditation, massage and reflexology, and support groups—do, in fact, make the cancer experience more bearable.

Less has been written about remission, a place where an increasing number of cancer patients reside. How do you cope with living between health and illness, with waiting for the potential return of an incurable condition? There is no shortage of books that offer "quick fixes" such as special diets or regimens of vitamins that supposedly prevent cancer or spark spontaneous cures. Some people sell products that "ensure" that the cancer that has "gone away" will never return. In this book we offer no such "quick fixes." There is no one path that leads to a life of perfect health and harmony. There is no singular way to live in the world as a cancer patient or, indeed, as a human being. Each person must choose his or her own path up the mountain.

What we can say with some degree of confidence is that engagement with the world through a variety of social and physical activities may not cure us of cancer, but such engagement can make life sweeter on the climb. As we climb higher up the mountain in search of greater understanding and wisdom, we eventually reach the mountaintop. At the summit, perhaps we'll find the satisfaction and comfort of knowing that we have managed our struggles to the best of our abilities, of knowing that our lives have been well lived.

SOURCES ON HAPPINESS AND WELL-BEING

1. Seligman, Martin. 2003. Authentic Happiness. New York: Nicholas Brealy Publishing.
2. Weissenstein, Michael. 2012. "Happiest People On Planet Live In Latin America, Gallup Poll Suggests." Associated Press, December 19.

CREDITS

Layout: Cornelia Knorr

Typesetting: Eva Feldmann

Cover: Andreas Reuel

Coverpicture: Thinkstock, Collection: iStock, TimHesterPhotography

Jacket: Eva Feldmann

Copy-editing: Jilian Evans